DIABETES AND WELLNESS: MOVEMENT, NUTRITION, FASTING, AND THE POWER OF OPTIMISM

Kenneth R. Ellis, M.S.

with Deb Ellis, Contributor

ISBN: 9798345858134 (paperback)
ISBN: 9798300423155 (hardback)

Imprint: Independently published

Also by Kenneth R. Ellis

7 Biblical Ways for Healthy Living:
Wisdom, Optimism, Kindness, Motivation,
Movement, Nutrition, and Stress Control

The Way of Wisdom for Diabetes:
Cope with Stress, Move More, Lose Weight and
Keep Hope Alive

Subscribe to the
Wisdom for Diabetes YouTube Channel
www.wisdomfordiabetes.org

CONTENTS

PART 2
COMMON SENSE GUIDELINES FOR LIVING WELL WITH DIABETES

Introduction

Wisdom's Value—The Skill for Optimistic Living

*"A good person gives life to others; the wise person
teaches others how to live* (Proverbs 11:30).

*"My son, do not forget my teaching, but keep my commands
in your heart, for they will prolong your life many years
and bring you peace and prosperity"* (Proverbs 3:1-2).

The foundation for these strategies is the **way of wisdom (skill for optimistic living), God's wisdom.** Success and victory come from God's wisdom. *"For the LORD gives wisdom; from his mouth come knowledge and understanding. He holds success (victory) in store for the upright"* (Proverbs 2:6-7). We all have available to us God's wisdom which is more precious than rubies. *"She is more precious than rubies; nothing you desire can compare with her. **Long life is in her right hand**"* (Proverbs 3:15). As you read through these strategies, you will see how vital and valuable the resource of **wisdom is or the power of optimism.** It could be called **the common-sense approach** that is not so common.

Victorious, optimistic living comes with hurdles and obstacles to overcome. So often, the compassion from others helps us through the difficulties. We can reflect upon a kind act with gratitude. Both are the way of wisdom. *"Your own soul is nourished when you are kind; it is destroyed when you are cruel"* (Proverbs 11:17). *"A bright look brings joy to the heart, and **good news gives health to the body**"* (Proverbs 15:30 NET). **Here is a personal example of mine, which happened in 1986 when I was thirty-three after having Type 1 Diabetes for about twenty-six years.**

Eyesight, Retinopathy, and a Compassionate Doctor

Almost forty years ago, as my wife and I and our two little boys were walking around a lake, I experienced a traumatic event. A dot appeared in my right eye. The dot kept growing. The beauty of the walkway and the lake were becoming a blur. By the time we returned to our car, I could barely see. I was experiencing a retinal hemorrhage into the vitreous of my eye. We had just moved to a new state and town. I knew no doctor for support. It was a Thursday, so the first thing I did was look for an ophthalmologist in the Yellow Pages. I went to see him the next day, but what he said didn't build my optimism. He said there is nothing we can do about it right now. The only thing you can do is pray. I told him I was already doing that.

I announced at church what had happened to me. Fortunately, a new friend in our church informed me of a specialist—an endocrinologist—Dr. Richard Hellman (in 2007-2008, he was president of the American Association of Clinical Endocrinologists). I saw him almost immediately. He then referred me to an ophthalmologist, Dr. Matthew Ziemianski. The retinal hemorrhage was distressing enough, but the shocking surprise that my health insurance company had just gone bankrupt made the situation an overwhelming burden! While sitting in the waiting room with my wife and two little boys, the doctor's nurse overheard a conversation I was having about my situation with another patient. She then informed the doctor.

So when I went into the doctor's office, he made a statement that I still get emotional about to this day, almost forty years later. He said his nurse had told him of my situation. Then he told me he would do laser treatment on my eyes without charge! He had seen me sitting in the waiting room with my wife and two little boys. I remember his words as if he spoke them yesterday: "Those boys need a father who can see. So, I'm going to do the surgeries without charge." He used the pan-retinal laser photocoagulation treatment in both eyes. When he said that, his words were the most meaningful and encouraging thing he could have said to me then. He did an excellent job with the laser treatment, helping me now have, thirty-eight years later, very good eyesight. His compassion and kindness were so significant that I was motivated to help others with support groups, diabetes educational seminars, and several books for more than thirty years! Let's all be compassionate to others and grateful for the kindness we've received. We will then make a positive difference in their lives and ours! *"A generous person will prosper (be healthy); whoever refreshes others will be refreshed"* (Proverbs 11:25). *"A cheerful look brings joy to the heart, and good news gives health to the body"* (Proverbs 15:30). My story introduces two of the seventeen ways to outsmart diabetes—#

6 (Focus on staying optimistic every day with gratitude, which is what I'm doing by reflecting on this story) and # 17 (Take advantage of opportunities to help others, which is what Dr. Ziemianski did for me).

Diabetes Management application: By doing the following 17 prime activities, you'll keep your safety harness on. Instead of letting diabetes do its devastating work in the background of your life, destroying your health, you will keep in control. So, let's start our day with seven vital guidelines.

Part 1
Diabetes and Wellness: Movement, Nutrition, Fasting, and The Power of Optimism—17 Wise Ways

CHAPTER ONE

Wise Ways to Stay in Control During the Morning

1 Keep Learning.

Ignorance is not bliss. When I went to see my Endocrinologist recently, I told him since I'm 69, I decided to try two new things. The first one was to donate blood. I tried to donate forty years ago but was not accepted since I had Type 1 Diabetes. But this time, I was accepted as long as I didn't have current diabetes complications and was in stable control. So my wife and I gave. And after doing so, I had a wonderful feeling about the good it would do.

The second thing I decided to do was look at the best-seller book list on Amazon for books under the category of Diabetes. When I saw the Diabetes Code was number 1, I decided to buy it. What a wise decision that was.

It is good to start the day knowing what Diabetes is. The better we understand, the better our choices will be. Instead of assuming what we need to do, we can know what to do. For example, someone asked me, since I have Type 1 Diabetes, when I would become Type 2. The fact is I will never become Type 2. Both types of Diabetes have similar lifestyles with meal plans and exercise but are dissimilar in many ways, like medications available for use. Both can use an effective therapy, but the results can reverse Type 2 Diabetes. Type 1s can use it to lose weight and cause their bodies to be more sensitive to insulin, making less needed. What is this therapy I discovered? Fasting and I found it in the information author and medical doctor Jason Fung wrote in the Diabetes Code.

The essential difference between the two types of Diabetes is the beta cells available in the pancreas to produce insulin. Type 1 is an autoimmune disease in which the body attacks and destroys the insulin-producing beta cells. Type 2 is a disease in which the beta cells keep producing to the point of stuffing the cells with glucose. That is how there becomes insulin resistance. Instead of being stored as glycogen, the body stores the excess glucose as fat. When fasting for sixteen hours, the body, after fourteen hours, uses the stored glucose, which is glycogen, and then converts to fat as its energy source. This means that the body begins to lose weight. So, it is imperative with either type to keep blood glucose as close to the normal range as possible and know that carbohydrates profoundly impact blood glucose levels and insulin production in people with Type 2 Diabetes. I give more information on metabolism with the fourth wise way of timing.

To view an explanation of how insulin moves glucose into cells, go to "Insulin, Glucose and You" at **https://www.youtube.com/watch?v=jqP9JmS_sKo.**

After knowing what Diabetes is, we need a plan to outsmart it daily! Almost everyone has a routine in the morning, but is it best for your health?

2 Have a health routine—a plan.

"Proper Prior Planning Prevents Pitifully Poor Performance.
People Don't Plan to Fail, They Fail to Plan.
Planning the Best Decisions Ahead of Time: Diligence"

"The wisdom of the prudent is to give thought to their ways, but the folly of fools is deception" (Proverbs 14:8).

"Sluggards do not plow in season; so at harvest time they look but find nothing" (Proverbs 20:4).

"The plans of the diligent lead to profit as surely as haste leads to poverty" (Proverbs 21:5).

Biblically, the basic meaning of diligence is planning.

People get out of bed in the morning and usually visit the restroom. What follows among people differs. Some have the simple habit of making their bed. Making your bed first thing in the morning is good, but there is a plan that is much more beneficial for those with diabetes! It is called checking your blood glucose or sugar level.

Planning keeps you free to control your diabetes. The desire to go back and do things differently happens in many situations. For example, have you ever locked your car and looked in to see your keys sitting on the seat? Even worse, what if you got locked into an ATM service room? A recent news headline was "Texas Police Make Odd Withdrawal from ATM: A Man Who Was Trapped Inside."[1] A contractor, who was changing the lock on the service room of an ATM, realized he had locked himself in the room. Unfortunately, he couldn't call anyone for help because he had left his cell phone in his truck.

What was he to do? He became very creative. People started receiving more than cash and a receipt at the ATM. They also got a handwritten note with their receipt—"Please Help. I'm stuck in here, and I don't have my phone. Please call my boss. At 210..." He did this for about two hours until one person finally took the message and called the police. "This is just a prank" is what most people thought, including the police, until someone behind the screen answered them. They broke the door down and freed the desperate man. A police officer said, "We have a once-in-a-lifetime situation that you'll probably never see or hear about again."

What lessons can we learn from this? First, giving thought to health is so important! How many times will I check my blood sugar today? Or how many steps will I take? How many calories will I eat, especially carbohydrates, since they directly impact my blood sugar levels? These are the things to think about first thing in the morning! The way of God's wisdom teaches the importance of planning, of not getting in a hurry, of not having to go back and do things differently. *"The plans of the diligent lead to profit as surely as haste leads to poverty"* (Proverbs 21: 5). *"Enthusiasm without knowledge is not good. If you act too quickly, you might make a mistake"* (Proverbs 19: 2). We all need to plan our days, build healthy habits, and to think before doing!

Watch: "Police Withdraw Man Trapped In Bank ATM" at https://www.youtube.com/watch?v=DDU7ibWTX9U.

3 Check your blood glucose level first thing in the morning!

Pricking your fingers hurts! So, why do it? (You experience less pain by pricking on the side of your finger, not the pad. Use a good lancet device like a "CareTouch," too.) Discovering your blood glucose will give you the information to make the best decision. What if you wake up with an elevated blood glucose of 185 or even 264? What should you do? Should you go ahead and eat breakfast? No, take a leisure walk instead, or avoid carbs for breakfast. What caused this? What was my blood glucose last night before going to bed? Do I have a cold starting? Did I eat a snack last night? Have relationship conflicts or financial stress? All these could be factors that cause elevated blood glucose in the morning. Where should your blood glucose be during the day? Here are some guidelines compared to normal numbers for those without diabetes.

Nighttime fasting and before breakfast: 70–130 mg/dl
Normal is less than 100 mg/dl
Before lunch, supper, and snacks: 70–130 mg/dl
Two hours after starting meals: 160 mg/dl or less
Normal is less than 140 mg/dl
Bedtime: 90–150 mg/dl
Normal is less than 120 mg/dl

http://www.joslin.org/docs/Pharm_Guideline_Graded.pdf

Many people have the good habit of checking their blood glucose in the morning—and then they are through checking for the day! However, research indicates that checking yourself more often than once daily will build greater self-management confidence and better glucose numbers. From this research, the A1c test results fell more than one point—7.3 to 6.2. (For more information on this topic, read pp. 31-37 in my book "The Way of Wisdom for Diabetes.")

4 Mimic God's design of the body with timing and carb counting— making the right time your habit.

"Timing Is (Almost) Everything"

Wisdom's way teaches the importance of timing:

> *"Anyone who refuses to work doesn't plow in the right season. When he looks for a crop at harvest time, he doesn't find it."* (Proverbs 20:4 NIrV)

> *"A person finds joy in giving an apt reply—and how good is a timely word!"* (Proverbs 15:23)

Since carbohydrates affect blood glucose, take your insulin before twenty to thirty minutes before breakfast or any meal (unless your blood glucose is below 70, then take it after the meal or if you order sitting in a restaurant. Wait until you see the food and eat carbs last). Novolog and Humalog become active within fifteen to twenty minutes and Fiasp and Lyumjev within five minutes. So, if you wake up at 163, take your insulin, walk and then eat breakfast, you could have low blood glucose. This happened with a friend of mine, and before he could get to breakfast, he was 38 mg/dl.

Mimic God's design of the body.

"We are fearfully and wonderfully made" (Psalm 139:14). God's wisdom teachings are for the health of one's whole body. *"Turn your ear to my words...for they are life to those who find them and health to one's whole body"* (Proverbs 4:20, 22). The Proverbs teaches principles like this one. *"Finish your outdoor work and get your fields ready; after that, build your house"* (Proverbs 24:27). The proverb teaches an important sequence concerning a person's financial welfare. If a person doesn't have the fields ready, there will not be a harvest for food to eat on the table. Building a house will not sustain a person with the nourishment needed. So, get your fields ready, so there can be a harvest and then have resources to build a house. A sequence of priority steps is needed for physical health too. So walk, eat, check blood glucose, take medications, and do so at just the right time! "You've got to be kidding?" No, we've already seen the importance of a sequence when starting the day.

We see a sequence in God's design of the body when we eat. What happens when we eat carbohydrates? Glucose is the result. First, the body transports Glucose with blood into the small intestine. Then, a step-by-step process begins to metabolize the Glucose for energy. In a sense, the body is counting the carbs you eat and initially responds by releasing stored-up insulin in secretory vesicles in the pancreas. Then it begins to manufacture the exact amount of insulin needed with the pancreas' beta cells.

Do you know you have some tiny but priceless islands? The Pancreas' Islets of Langerhans (about 1 million of them) are the priceless islands. They are priceless because, within each one, you have about two thousand beta cells and alpha cells (producing the hormone glucagon). Within the beta cells, the hormone insulin is manufactured in a multi-step process; the word insulin is from a Latin root word meaning island. And insulin is produced in the Islets of Langerhans. "These are capable of measuring the blood glucose level within seconds with an accuracy to within 2 mg/dl (0.1 mmol/1) to determine the quantity of insulin needed," writes Dr. Richard Beaser of the Joslin Diabetes Center.[2] Especially when we eat carbohydrates, glucose levels rise. Stored insulin then deploys rapidly, which is called phase 1 insulin release. Unfortunately, most people with Type 2 diabetes have an impaired phase 1 release of insulin. This can cause a high blood glucose reading after a meal and a low hypoglycemic episode several hours later with too much insulin in circulation.

Insulin is a multifaceted hormone capable of doing several functions, and here are some of them. Insulin aids glucose entry into cells for energy storage and heat production. Since its discovery 100 years ago, this has been the focus of insulin. When Banting and Best discovered insulin, doctors used it for patients needing glucose control. And even the term "diabetes (siphon Greek), mellitus (sweet Latin)" evokes the "honey urine that attracts ants" idea recognized since antiquity but first documented by Thomas Willis in 1674. With the use of insulin, patients and healthcare providers focus on Blood sugar control to prevent complications. This has been my focus as a person with Type 1 Diabetes for sixty-four+ years, and it brings life instead of death for Type 1s.

People newly diagnosed with diabetes can be confused about what to eat and what not to eat. One man said, *"My doctor told me about the importance of a healthy meal plan, which—as near as I can tell—means I'm only allowed to eat birdseed all day."* At one time, it was almost that bad. Before 1921, people took drastic measures to continue to breathe with no quality of life. In 1919, Dr. Frederick Allen published Total Dietary Regulation in the Treatment of Diabetes, citing detailed case records of 76 of the 100 diabetes patients he observed—called Type 1 patients today! His treatment for them was to start with an extremely low-carbohydrate diet and gradually increase to the renal threshold, or the level of blood glucose above which the kidneys fail to reabsorb—and thus spill—glucose into the urine. The renal threshold is about 180 mg/dl. What this meant for most people was living on a diet plan or "starvation therapy" of very little food per day. They virtually eliminated carbs from their diet. So we can summarize the treatment as eat less, be hungrier!

People on this therapy were described by Dr. Elliott Joslin with the first ten verses of Ezekiel 37 as the "Valley of Dry Bones," referring to Ezekiel's description of the Jewish exiles from Judea to Babylon. *"Can these bones live?....I will cause breath to enter you so you will come to life. I will put muscles on you and flesh on you and cover you with skin. Then I will put breath in you so you will come to life"* (Ezekiel 37:1ff). These Jews were people who had everything taken from them—their homes, their way of life, their worship. They were taken hundreds of miles away without any prospects of returning, of their lives turning back to how they used to be. They were in despair, without any hope of a joyful life.

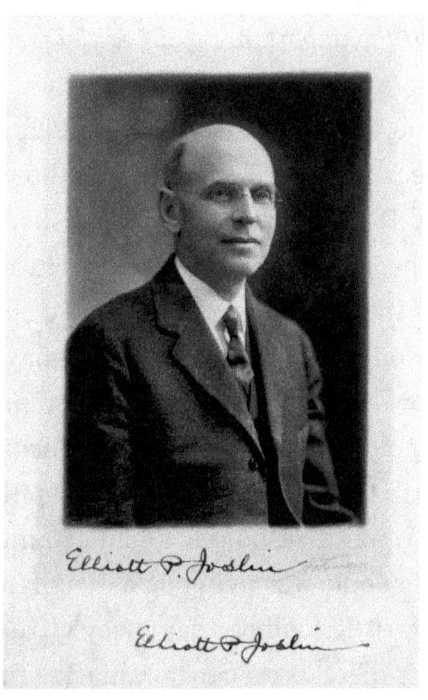

Dr. E. P. Joslin of Boston was one of the first doctors to receive insulin for his patients. Photo courtesy of The Thomas Fisher Rare Book Library, University of Toronto.

Diabetes was taking hope and life and living well from them. Dr. Joslin saw the "valley of dry bones" among these people with diabetes, who were gradually starving to death. In 1922, his description changed because insulin restored them to a healthier life. One boy named J. L. weighed fifteen pounds on December 15, 1922, at the age of three, but after being on insulin for just two months, he weighed twenty-nine pounds. Dr. Joslin writes, "By Christmas of 1922, I had witnessed so many near resurrections that I realized I was seeing enacted before my eyes Ezekiel's vision of the valley of dry bones.... It still remains a wonder that this limpid liquid (insulin) injected under the skin two times a day can metamorphosize a baby, child or frail adult or old man or woman to their nearly normal counterparts."[3]

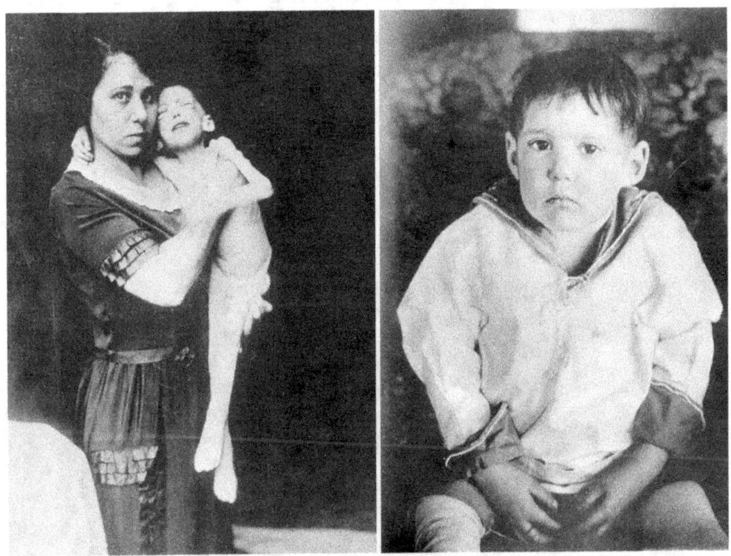

Three-year-old J. L. before insulin. J.L. two months later, on insulin. Photo courtesy of Eli Lilly and Company Archives.

Dr. Banting was a surgeon during World War 1. While in the battle zone, shrapnel wounded his right forearm. They removed it and applied a tourniquet above his elbow. He then continued to work on the injured for seventeen hours. This is the kind of character he had! After his time in World War 1, he became a demonstrator in surgery and anatomy at the University of Western Ontario. In this role, he had to talk to medical students about the pancreas, which led him to read about the islets of Langerhans in a medical journal. One night, as he prepared for a lecture on carbohydrate metabolism, he read a November 1920 issue of Surgery, Gynaecology and Obstetrics. The article's title was "The Relation of the Islets of Langerhans to Diabetes with Special Reference to Cases of Pancreatic Lithiasis." It was so intriguing that he couldn't get to sleep that night. That night at about 2 a.m., after reading the article, he got up and wrote, "trying to isolate the internal secretion" of dogs' pancreatic ducts. This led him and his assistant, Charles Best, to discover insulin.[4]

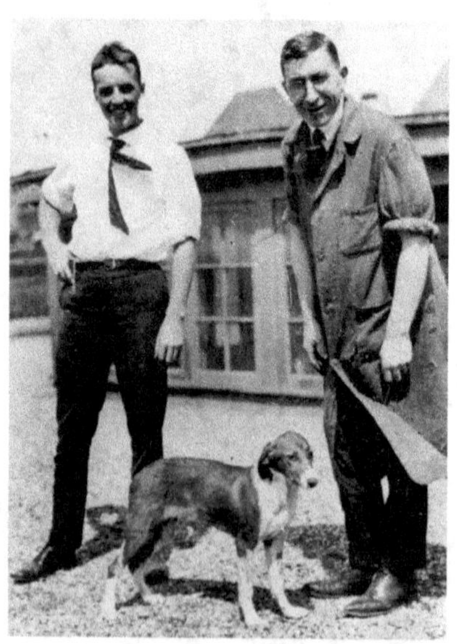

Charles Best and Dr. Frederick Banting, discoverers of insulin.
Photo courtesy of The Thomas Fisher Rare
Book Library, University of Toronto

His idea was to extract a substance from the islets, later known as insulin, using the lab at Toronto University. He and a graduate assistant, Charles Best, used lab dogs, dog pound dogs, and even strays that summer for their experiments. Dr. Frederick Banting and Charles Best tied off the pancreas duct in dogs and discovered insulin on July 27, 1921.

When Banting and Best discovered insulin, the first person to receive a large, unrefined dose was a dying fourteen-year-old boy named Leonard Thompson. He had lived for two years on the "under-nutrition, starvation" therapy that the leading diabetologist recommended—Dr. Frederick Allen. He lived another fifteen years with insulin injections but with a lack of self-control. His behavior contributed to his short life.[5]

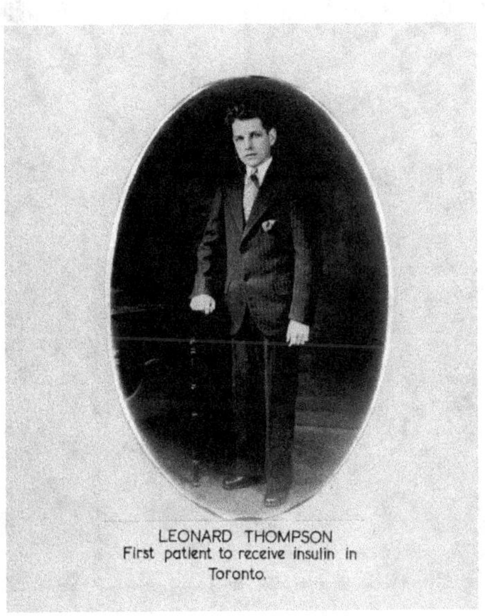

Leonard Thompson first person given insulin.
Photo courtesy of The Thomas Fisher Rare
Book Library, University of Toronto.

On the other hand, Teddy Ryder was five years old and weighed twenty-six pounds when Dr. Banting gave him his first life-saving dose of insulin. When Teddy's uncle, Dr. Mortin Ryder, asked for insulin for his nephew in the summer of 1922, Dr. Banting suggested that he write again in September. The supply was unstable and impure. Dr. Ryder replied, "Teddy won't be alive in September."

So, Dr. Banting decided to accept him as a patient. Teddy had loving people who cared about him, and from them, he learned to be motivated to take care of himself. He lived for seventy years with daily insulin injections. He died in 1993 at seventy-six, the last of the original group of Dr. Banting's patients.

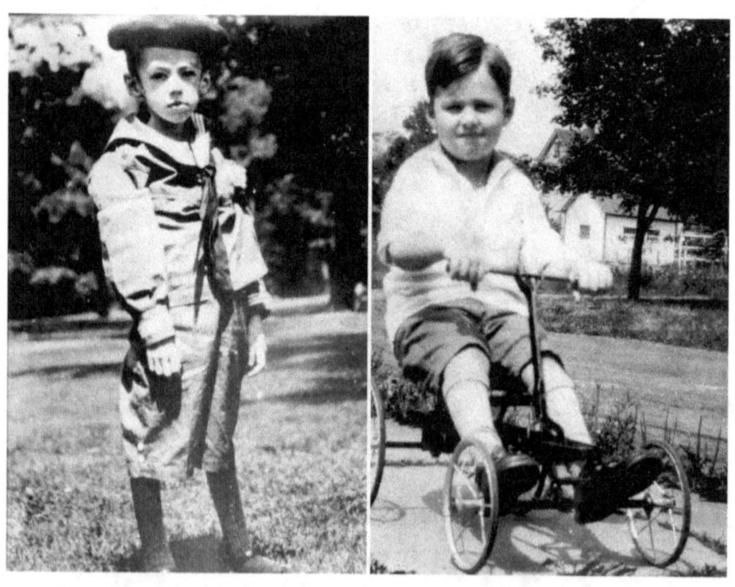

Teddy Ryder before insulin and one-year after insulin.
Photo courtesy of The Thomas Fisher Rare
Book Library, University of Toronto.

Dr. Allen returns from Toronto after visiting Dr. Banting at his treatment clinic, and this is what happened. "Diabetics who had not been out of bed for weeks began to trail weakly about, clinging to walls and furniture. It was a resurrection. When he appeared through the open doorway, he caught the full beseeching of a hundred pairs of eyes," writes nurse Margate Kienast. His voice curiously mingled concern for his patients with excitement that he tried his best not to betray. "I think," he said, "I think we have something for you."

So what became the treatment and management of Type 1 & 2 diabetes for decades? Insulin! Now we see these ways to manage Type 2 diabetes—improved diet, regular exercise, healthy weight, medications to control blood sugar, and self-management through lifestyle. I am so thankful for insulin. Since I was diagnosed with diabetes at the age of seven and started on insulin immediately, it has given me sixty-four+ years of a good life. If you have Type 1 Diabetes, you too should be thankful for insulin, giving you hope for a great life! However, this does not address the core issue of Type 2 Diabetes, which we will look at in a few pages.

Here is another function of insulin. Insulin enhances the process by which cells make proteins and cell growth. Insulin increases protein synthesis because insulin is one of the anabolic (growth and building) hormones along with growth hormone in the body. Insulin builds! Its main action is "opening" the cells so glucose can enter. Insulin also promotes protein synthesis by aiding the amino acids' entry into cells. Amino acids are molecules that combine to form proteins. Amino acids and proteins are the building blocks of life.[6]

But too much insulin affects people with insulin resistance and eventually Type 2 Diabetes. The liver stockpiles glucose into glycogen. But the liver has its limits for glycogen storage. Once that limit is reached, the overflow in glucose triggers another insulin function. It starts the liver with the excess glucose into fat through de novo lipogenesis (DNL). De novo (from new) and lipogenesis (making new fat), so De novo lipogenesis means "to make new fat." Insulin turns excess glucose into new fat in the form of triglyceride molecules. This new fat is stored in fat cells that the body can use for energy.

Insulin Resistance and Hyperinsulinemia occur when the cells are already full of glucose and the glucose-to-fat conversion starts. According to Dr. Jason Fung, this results in more stored fat or fatty liver. Insulin will also reduce fat movement. So where do you want to move fat? Out of the organs and fat around organs.[7]

Your body also can self-heal by not trying to eat when you are ill. In other words, your body goes into a fasting state. A fasting state can be healthy for losing weight and cutting back on the need for more insulin.

Jesus fasted. *"After fasting forty days and forty nights, he was hungry"* Matthew 4:2. Jesus was very weak, and Satan knew he was. This is when he tempted him by saying to turn stones into bread. But Jesus demonstrated that even in his condition, he could resist the temptation to use his powers in a self-centered way. But the point is Jesus fasted. Here is what other noteworthy people from history have said about fasting. "Instead of using medicine, better fast today," said Plutarch. "I fast for greater physical and mental efficiency," said Plato. Benjamin

Franklin wrote, "The best of all medicines is resting and fasting." "Everyone has a doctor in him; we just have to help him in his work. The natural healing force within each one of us is the greatest force in getting well...to eat when you are sick, is to feed your sickness," said Hippocrates.

To give you the full perspective on insulin's primary function to analyze, here is the traditional explanation. "Produced in the pancreas, insulin is a very special type of protein made for a very special and specific function critical to diabetes. Working throughout the body, affecting all cell types, insulin's main purpose is to stimulate cells to take up glucose from the bloodstream and transport this glucose into the cell's interior. To do this, cells must have receptors on their surfaces that interact with insulin, creating openings in the cell wall to allow passage of glucose into the cell. Think of a cell as a tiny fortified city on the bank of a busy river and imagine that the supplies for this city are delivered by ships passing through locked gates. In the body, the bloodstream is like the river that carries supplies to the cell wall and it is insulin that serves as the key that unlocks the gate, allowing the supplies, in this case, glucose, to enter the cell once the gate is opened. Diabetes develops when insufficient glucose enters the cell to meet the cell's energy needs and accumulates in the bloodstream. Two conditions must be met to provide adequate glucose for the cell; there must be enough insulin keys to open the gates, and, very importantly, the locks on these gates must work properly. Correspondingly, there are two types of diabetes, type I in which the insulin keys are lacking and type II in which the insulin receptors, or locks, malfunction."[8]

Another aspect of Type 2 diabetes involves the small intestine and what are known as incretin hormones. During a meal, the small intestine absorbs glucose, delivering the glucose to the blood. In response to glucose absorption, two incretin hormones are secreted. The intestine releases glucagon-like peptide GLP-1 and glucose-dependent insulin atrophic polypeptide GIP. They signal increased levels of glucose which then causes the secretion of insulin from the beta cells of the pancreas.[9]

With diabetes, the communication lines between these incretin hormones to the beta cells are impaired. An enzyme DPP-4 gets in the way of the GLP-1, causing releasing of insulin to end too quickly. The GLP-1 also suppresses the release of the hormone glucagon, which releases stored glucose or glycogen in the liver. Also, GLP-1 slows the process of metabolizing food. Since the GLP-1 hormone can become less effective in Type 2 Diabetes, there are now medications that help make the GLP-1 hormone more effective like Trulicity, Victoza, and Bydureon taken by injection. Also Ozempic® (semaglutide) and Mounjaro (tirzepatide) another medication in this category which I explain for weight loss in **#11—Eat carbs last as you slowly eat.** Watch "Trulicity (Dulaglutide). What does it do and how do I use it?" at **https://www.youtube.com/watch?v=x_8mfR1Jkes** There are also DPP-4 inhibitors like Januvia and Onglyza.

Watch: "DPP-4 Inhibitors in Action" at **https://www.youtube.com/watch?v=Ixk_wDPtPfk**

So how can we mimic the design of the body? What is the body doing when we eat? Measures glucose amounts. Glucose comes from carbohydrates. So, we should count our carbohydrate intake—count carbs, as well as know what our blood glucose level is. The fewer carbs you eat results in less stimulation of insulin, which causes more fat storage. So it would help to eat fewer carbs per day, under a hundred grams or even less. As a Type 1, I inject insulin. Using short-acting insulin like Humalog and Novolog, (I am now using Fiasp which takes less than five minutes to become active.) I take it about fifteen minutes before eating the calculated number of carbs I plan to eat. I do this if my blood glucose is over 120 mg/dl. If my blood glucose is less than 100, I take the insulin right before my first bite, and if it is 70 mg/dl, I wait about twenty minutes into the meal. Yes, timing is important. *"There is a time for everything, and a season for every activity under the heavens"* (Ecclesiastes 3:1).

5 Eat breakfast and all meals with fewer carbs and more protein and vegetables.

Eat fewer carbohydrates for every meal.
Portion control is the principle.

**"Wise People Keep Themselves Under Control:
Portion Control, Healthy Choices, and Self-Control"**

"If you find honey, eat just enough. If you eat too much of it, you will throw up" (Proverbs 25:16 NIrV).

"It is not good to eat too much honey, nor does it bring you honor to brag about yourself" (Proverbs 25:27 NCV).

Robert Buynak, M.D., in his book "Dr. Buynak's 1-2-3 Diabetes Diet," gives an accurate formula for determining how many calories to eat each day and maintaining your current weight. The formula is current weight x 11 = daily calories. For example, your weight is 230 pounds x 11 = 2500 calories per day. Since it takes 3500 calories to equal one pound, if you subtract 500 calories per day, you should lose one pound per week. That is, until you reach a plateau of loss. If that happens, you can always try # 14 Intermittent Fasting. How many of those calories should be carbohydrates? The Joslin Diabetes Deskbook recommends 40 % of the 2000 calories as carbohydrates, 800 calories (800/4 calories per gram), or 200 grams of carbohydrate per day.

Since carbohydrates directly affect blood glucose levels, the less you eat, the better your blood glucose control will be. What is the ideal amount of carbohydrates to eat per day? Some advocates of a low-carb meal plan really mean low-carb! Some suggest up to 12 to 15 grams of carbs per meal, comparable to eating just one slice of bread. For the day, they suggest no more than 50 grams. If that is what it takes to keep blood glucose in control, do it! But if you can eat more, maintain blood glucose levels near normal, and lose weight, do it! I usually eat about 15-20 grams for breakfast and 30-35 grams for dinner (lunch) and supper, and an additional 12-15 for snacks during the day (or 90-110 grams per day, which equals 27 % carbs for my weight of 145 lbs.). To determine the grams of carbohydrates in various foods, go to **www.calorieking.com**. Using the FreeStyle Libre continuous glucose monitoring system, I've been above 140 mg/dl less than 20 % of the time with a 105-110 average.

The carbohydrates to eat should raise blood glucose levels the least. Numbers have been assigned based on research on how fast a particular carbohydrate will make blood glucose rise in two hours compared to an equal quantity of pure glucose. Researchers compared all carbohydrates to glucose, giving the baseline number 100. The smaller the number is, the better the results will be for maintaining good blood glucose levels. The glycemic load (GL) number is for the "typical" serving. The result of each food number they give at **www.glycemicindex. com.** They put the results into three categories based on the glycemic index number. The following list has the best carbohydrates to eat with the least effect on blood glucose:

Low: 55 and under (<10 GL). Examples include apple, fresh, medium (38 GI, 6 GL, 4 oz, 15 Carb grams), banana, fresh, medium (52 GI, 12 GL, 4 oz, 24 Carb grams), black beans, cooked (30 GI, 7 GL, 4/5 cup, 23 Carb grams), black-eyed peas, canned (42 GI, 7 GL, 2/3 cup, 17 Carb grams), brown rice, cooked (50 GI, 16 GL, 1 cup, 33 Carb grams), carrots, peeled, cooked (49 GI, 2 GL, ½ cup, 5 Carb grams), carrots, raw (47 GI, 3 GL, 1 medium, 6 Carb grams), cherries, fresh (22 GI, 3 GL, 18 cherries, 12 Carb grams), chickpeas or garbanzo beans, canned (42 GI, 9 GL, 2/3 cup, 22 Carb grams), French green beans, cooked (0 GI, 0 GL, ½ cup, 0 Carb grams), grapefruit, fresh, medium (25 GI, 3 GL, 1 half, 11 Carb grams), grapes, green, fresh (46 GI, 8 GL, ¾ cup, 18 Carb grams), green peas (48 GI, 3 GL, 1/3 cup, 7 Carb grams), honey (55 GI, 10 GL, 1 Tbsp, 18 Carb grams), kidney beans, canned (52 GI, 9 GL, 2/3 cup, 17 Carb grams), kidney beans, cooked (23 GI, 6 GL, 2/3 cup, 25 Carb grams), 28, 7), lentils, brown, cooked (29 GI, 5 GL, ¾ cup, 18 Carb grams), lentils, red, cooked, (26 GI, 5 GL, ¾ cup, 18 Carb grams), lima beans, baby, frozen (32 GI, 10 GL, ¾ cup 30 Carb grams), navy beans, canned (38 GI, 12 GL, 5 oz, 31 Carb grams), peach, fresh, large (42 GI, 5 GL, 4 oz, 11 Carb grams), peanuts (14 GI, 1 GL, 1.75 oz, 6 Carb grams), pear halves, canned in natural juice (43 GI, 5 GL, ½ cup, 13 Carb grams), pear, fresh (38 GI, 4 GL, 4 oz, 11 Carb grams), peas, green, frozen, cooked (48 GI, 3 GL, ½ cup, 7 Carb grams), pinto beans, canned (45 GI, 10 GL, 2/3 cup, 22 Carb grams), pinto beans, dried, cooked (39 GI, 10 GL, ¾ cup, 26 Carb grams), rolled oats (42 GI, 9 GL, 1 cup, 21 Carb grams), seeded rye bread (55 GI, 7 GL, 1 oz, 13 Carb grams), sourdough rye (48 GI, 6 GL, 1 oz, 12 Carb grams), sourdough wheat (54 GI, 8 GL, 1 oz, 14 Carb grams), strawberries, fresh (40 GI, 1 GL, 4 oz, 3 Carb grams), sweet corn, whole kernel, canned, diet-pack, drained (46 GI, 13 GL, 1 cup, 28 Carb grams), sweet potato, cooked (44 GI, 11 GL, 5 oz, 25 Carb grams), tomato, chopped (28 GI, 2 GL, 1 cup, 8 Carb grams).[10]

For a good explanation of carbohydrates, watch "How do carbohydrates impact your health?—Richard J. Wood" at **https://www.youtube.com/watch?v=wxzc_2c6GMg**

By eating fewer carbohydrates per meal, you should eat **more vegetables and protein.** First, let's notice a way to increase eating vegetables for your health benefit.

What would happen if you ate a salad before each meal? Would it affect how much you would eat for the entire meal? Forty-two women participated in a study conducted by the Department of Nutritional Sciences of Penn State University to research that very idea. They gave several lunch options for each lunch. The control condition was not to eat a salad before the meal's main course, pasta. They were to eat as much pasta as they desired, and the researchers measured the amount they ate.

Other lunch options were various sizes and energy densities of salads. The participants were required to eat the salads before the main course. The portion size of the salads used was either 150 grams or 300 grams of weight. The researchers changed the energy density of the salad by changing the dressing and cheese. The salad was smaller when more weight was taken by the dressing or cheese used, bringing the weight to either 150 grams or 300 grams, but with less lettuce or vegetables. For example, the 150-gram salad came with three levels of total calories: fifty, one hundred, or two hundred calories. If it were the low-energy-density salad, it would equal about three cups of salad with a very light dressing. The 300-gram salad came with the same calculations (0.33, 0.67, or 1.33 kcal/g, or one hundred, two hundred, or four hundred total calories).[11]

According to this study, if you want to control or lose weight, eat a salad without high-calorie dressings or cheese before your main course at dinner or supper. When they ate low-energy-density salads—the salads that pack more volume of food on the plate or in the bowl but with fewer calories—they ate less food during the main course of pasta. In other words, starting a meal with this type of salad enhances satiety or the feeling of being full and thus reduces the amount of calories eaten during the main course.

The study further determined that a salad for weight loss is an effective strategy when a large portion is eaten before meals. For the smaller salad of 150 grams, with a low-calorie dressing, 7 percent less was eaten for the main course; and for the 300-gram salad, it was 12 percent. This practical application is something you can easily incorporate into your daily routine. For instance, you can take the prepackaged salads (like romaine) and make a salad with two servings, or three cups, which is thirty calories; and add a serving of low-calorie vinaigrette dressing, which is another thirty calories, for a grand total of sixty calories.

According to the research, if you use calorie-rich dressings like blue cheese, which has seventy-six calories and 8 grams of fat per serving, or Thousand Island dressing, which has sixty calories and almost 6 grams of fat, you will eat more for the main course. When two salads with the same number of calories were compared, it was found that meal intake decreased when a large portion of the lower-energy-density salad was consumed, and meal intake increased with the smaller portion of the energy-dense salad.

The message is clear—leave off the rich dressings! Use the low-calorie dressings. It's up to you to make healthier choices. Use dressings like vinaigrette or the wide assortment of Walden Farms no-calorie dressings—https://www.waldenfarms.com/—and have more salad! One person in our diabetes support group began concentrating on eating more salad with the Walden Farms dressings. Tremendous benefits for her blood glucose levels resulted, going from an A1c of 12.4 (309 BG average) to an 8.2 A1c (189 BG average). The power to improve your health is in your hands. Eat more salad!

Second, half your body weight is the recommended number of grams of protein you should eat daily. The Joslin Diabetes

Deskbook lists several benefits of eating more protein, such as a sensation of fullness, maintaining muscle mass while losing weight, better uptake of glucose by muscles, and reducing the spike up of blood glucose after meals.[12] Eat healthy protein. Think of eating fish, turkey, and chicken. We've used many delicious low-carb chicken recipes from Paleo Magazine.

The following from Calorieking.com are the calorie values of one ounce of meat. The amount of protein per ounce is about 7 to 8 grams. Roasted turkey breast, without skin, has 38 calories. Cooked pink salmon has 42 calories. White tuna (Albacore), canned in water and drained, has 36 calories. Rotisserie chicken breast, without skin, with original seasoning, has 42 calories. 96% Fat-free ham, sliced, has 31 calories. Now notice the contrast of highly concentrated saturated fat protein like sausage and ground beef. Fresh beef sausage, cooked, has 94 calories. Ground beef, 95% lean, 5% fat, pan-browned, has 55 calories. Ground beef, 80% lean, 20% fat, pan-browned, has 77 calories. For each ounce of sausage, you can eat three ounces of fat-free ham or turkey breast. It is obvious which one will fill you up. I'm choosing the fat-free ham or turkey breast. What about you?

6 Focus on staying optimistic every day with gratitude.

One of the first things to do to start the day is to jot down good things that happened the previous day. (You could do this in the evening before bed as sleep preparation too.) Then give thanks to God for them. Looking at the brighter side of life is the principle.

"Count Your Blessings, and You Will Show a
Profit. Have the Attitude of Gratitude. Look on
the Brighter Side of Life—The Good News."

---

*"Whoever seeks good finds favor, but evil comes
to one who searches for it."* (Proverbs 11:27).

*"A cheerful look brings joy to your heart. And good
news gives health to your body"* (Proverbs 15:30).

*"A cheerful heart makes you healthy. But a broken
spirit dries you up"* (Proverbs 17:22 NIrV).

*"Hearing good news from a land far away is like drinking
cold water when you are tired"* (Proverbs 25:25 NIrV).

Health benefits from the practice of gratitude have been shown from extensive scientific research by Robert Emmons, Ph.D., when at the University of California at Davis, by researchers at the University of Pittsburgh, University of Manchester, University of Pennsylvania, and the University of Michigan and more. From this research, a practice of gratitude contributes to sleeping better, exercising more, reducing levels of the stress hormone cortisol, feeling more optimistic and connected with others. Also, people who practice gratitude have better compliance or adherence to a meal plan and taking their medications.[13]

Watch: "Robert Emmons: What Good is Gratitude?"
at Robert Emmons: What Good Is Gratitude?
https://www.youtube.com/watch?v=aRV8AhCntXc

Watch: "Yale's Most Popular Class Is Teaching Students How To Lead Happier Lives | NBC Nightly News" at **https://www.youtube.com/watch?v=tarn7tJk5NE**

Here are three ways to practice gratitude. Have you ever had thoughts like these? I have. "It happens over and over. Yesterday, for example, I followed my prescribed meal plan almost perfectly, and I even skipped dinner. So I woke up this morning, and my blood sugar was 300. This is ridiculous. Why should I bother even trying."

It's easy to complain about the bad things happening in our lives, but it takes more effort to think about the good things. When we consider all the things available today to help manage diabetes, compared to how it's been in the past, we can put those things on a "Feel Good Page" and be thankful. Medications like Jardiance; new insights into nutrition, fasting, and movement; and new tools like insulin pens, insulin pumps, and glucose monitors you can list on the "Feel Good Page." The way of wisdom teaches us to focus on that page!

"Pleasant words are like honey. They are sweet to the spirit and bring healing to the body." (Proverbs 16:24).

"He who seeks good finds goodwill, but evil comes to him who searches for it" (Proverbs 11:27).

The first point is to list what is good on your "Feel Good Page." Make sure you list the seemingly insignificant trivial things too. You shouldn't take them for granted. We should look for minor things. Count them. List them. Pray about them. For example, we can have a good day using our **hands** in the yard or garden or at our computer, **see** the beauty of flowers, and enjoy the **aroma** and **taste** of delicious food with gratitude! To see, walk, taste, feel, "eat, as well as have a home," bed, clothes, family, and friends are the little things we should appreciate and not take for granted!

Watch: "After Growing Up Homeless, Boy Is Over The Moon For His New Bed | NBC Nightly News" **https://www.youtube.com/watch?v=vJ0eC88Km-0**

Secondly, talk to yourself in a positive, encouraging, and reaffirming way. Dr. Gary Arsham, a medical doctor with Type 1 Diabetes for more than sixty years, wrote this. "You are the best available source of support for living well with diabetes. You are always there, and you know yourself well; no one else can take care of you as well as you can." Take to heart those words and then add these affirmations from Dr. Richard Beaser of the Joslin Diabetes Center. "I am a strong and self-assured individual, so that when monitoring or scheduling require-ments affect my activities with others, I handle my needs without giving in to group pressures. I feel comfortable with and am able to educate those around me about why I need to frequently check and count my carbohydrates. I feel comfortable in my ability to make appropriate adaptations so that I can participate in social activities that I enjoy."

So after listing good things on your "Feel Good Page" and talking to yourself in a positive, affirming way, add this third way to develop more gratitude—comparing yourself to others. Have you ever compared yourself with others? If you were to do so, what would be the best way to do it? Saying, "I wish I were like so-and-so," or saying, "I wish I was healthier, wealthier, and wiser like so-and-so." If you practice this approach, it can bring envy or resentment instead of gratitude. Better to say, "I'm thankful or glad I'm not like so and so." For example, when I was recovering from surgery, I was in a hospital wing for only people with diabetes.

A twenty-seven-year-old blind patient was in the room next to me. He blamed everyone for his situation except himself. Instead of using the click button at his bed to call a nurse, he would rant and rave like a madman. Sometimes he would also bang on the wall while ranting, which was the wall that separated our rooms. He had been in and out of the hospital with diabetic ketoacidosis DKA, which is a condition that results from the lack of insulin for an extended period. This results in a toxic way of metabolizing food for energy, resulting in a concentration of free fatty acids, dehydration, and loss of fluid which brings fewer electrolytes like potassium, chloride, and sodium and an increase in counter-regulatory hormones like glucagon and cortisol. I believe this did not have to happen to him if he had just learned to use the principles we've examined. So this is the comparison: "I'm glad I'm not like this twenty-seven-year-old, being bitter and blaming others for his diabetes self-management."

You could make the same type of comparison with James Havens. Doctors diagnosed James with diabetes in 1914. He became the first American to receive insulin on May 22, 1922! To see the whole picture of how few resources were available to live with Type 1 Diabetes, read his story in the second part of this book.

Regarding resource devices, the following is an example of devices that directly relate to diabetes management and should be appreciated. The good news is glucose meters to check what our glucose levels are. For my first twenty-one years with diabetes, glucose meters did not exist! Now with a tiny amount of blood, we can check glucose levels with results in five to six seconds. But it hasn't always been that way! My first glucose meter was an Ames I purchased in the summer of 1981. You had to be near a sink and have a large drop of blood to use it. You then placed the blood on the strip, pushed a button on the meter, and a one-minute countdown would start. Once a minute had elapsed, I would apply a high-pressure dose of water from a small bottle to the strip, washing away what blood had not absorbed into the strip. The strip was then ready to be inserted into the meter for another one-minute countdown. Finally, after following these procedures, which took over two minutes, the result would be displayed. Do you see why the Way of Wisdom principle of good news and gratitude applies to what we have available today? *"A cheerful look brings joy to your heart. And good news gives health to your body"* (Proverbs 15:30 NIrV).

Now more innovative ways to check blood glucose are available—continuous glucose monitoring systems. No finger pricks with a lancet are required. Instead, a painless scan is all that is needed to know what your blood glucose is. For example, Dexcom, Medtronic, and Abbott offer user-friendly systems. Abbott calls theirs The Freestyle Libre system. It uses a scanning device called a Reader or an app for a smartphone. All you have to do is place it about one inch over a sensor attached to the back of your arm. The Reader then scans from the sensor, which lasts for fourteen days, what your blood glucose level is. The reading is from the interstitial fluid, not directly from the blood.

The sensor, about the size of two stacked quarters, is easily attached to the back of your arm. A tiny filament remains just under the skin in the arm's interstitial fluid (We've all heard our bodies are composed of about 55-60% fluid). Glucose first enters the bloodstream before it seeps into the interstitial fluid. So, there is a short lag between the glucose readings from continuous monitoring systems and a blood glucose meter. Using the trend arrow on the Reader, whether it points up or down, indicates that your blood glucose is currently a little higher or lower than the glucose number shown. I enthusiastically recommend these devices for your use! If you are low or high, the Reader will recommend you do a blood glucose meter check. We can list these devices on our "Feel Good Page." For more information, go to **https://freestylelibre.us/**

Watch: at Youtube "See More, Manage Better"
https://www.youtube.com/watch?v=-q8ixdYZCco&t=47s

7 Move Often Throughout the Day: Stand Up (at least 32 times a day), Strengthen Up, and Stretch Out

"Don't Just Sit There, Keep Moving"

*"Go to the ant, you sluggard; consider its ways
and be wise! It has no commander, no overseer or
ruler, yet it stores its provisions in summer and
gathers its food at harvest"* (Proverbs 6:6–8).

*"From the fruit of their lips people are filled
with good things, and the work of their hands
brings them reward"* (Proverbs 12:14).

*"All hard work pays off. But if all you do is talk,
you will be poor"* (Proverbs 14:23 NIrV).

*"Ants are creatures of little strength, yet they store
up their food in the summer"* (Proverbs 30:25).

Remember that when Solomon wrote these proverbs, most work involved manual labor. The principle is to move often throughout the day.

Move often is also good news for blood glucose control. Just getting up out of our chairs and leisurely walking for a couple of minutes every thirty minutes can make the difference. Research indicates that postprandial (after a meal) glucose is lowered from potential highs by half. Not only are glucose high levels reduced, but exercise also lowers cholesterol and triglycerides, and levels of lipoprotein lipase increase. This enzyme aids in the breakdown of fat in the bloodstream.

More good news comes from a study that analyzed the difference a fifteen-minute leisure walk after a meal would make on blood glucose levels compared to just sitting. Picture your blood glucose as a daunting ice-capped mountain peak by sitting compared to an image of safe, green rolling hills by walking. By just sitting, you will see your blood sugars climb higher and higher to the peak, but walking can cut the rise in half. So, I've learned to take a short walk after a meal rather than sit.

And here is an additional benefit. Walking reduces insulin levels and makes your muscles more sensitive to insulin. It takes tremendous exercise to burn seventy calories, the amount in a slice of bread. So, that is not why exercise benefits better health; instead, it cuts back on insulin resistance. When you take a walk for a few minutes, your body becomes more sensitive to insulin for the time you are walking and up to the following 48 hours.

How long can you breathe before becoming fatigued? Have you ever thought about that? As you read this, you are still breathing. You aren't exhausted, and that is because of the abundance of mitochondria in the muscle cells. They are tiny energy producers. The muscles with the most mitochondria, like the heart, have a slow contraction speed and slow twitch conduction, not fast like your hand muscles have. You can exhaust your hand muscles by using them too much. Your breathing muscles' activity is aerobic because the mitochondria aid the cells as tiny energy producers, providing oxygen and fatigue resistance. So, when we start walking, the leg muscles do not fatigue because they are abundant with mitochondria. When you walk, there is a response for less insulin needed, which can last for up to 48 hours. Insulin resistance reverses, and blood sugar comes down.[14]

When I walk, I speed up my pace and even jog for half a block. This is called **interval training** or intermittently speeding up the pace. People with Type 2 Diabetes who usually walked 10,000 steps daily participated in a twelve-week study of picking up the pace for part of their daily steps. They walked their typical 10,000 steps but increased their speed for part of their walks. As a result, they experienced an increase in how well their insulin worked—insulin sensitivity. Dr. Colberg, an exercise expert with Type 1 Diabetes, mentions several good benefits of this exercise, such as burning more fat and glucose, improving blood glucose control, strengthening the heart, and extending the calorie-burning power of muscles after workouts.[15]

For a good formula to determine intensity using your heart rate, look at the article "Exercise Intensity: How to Measure It" by the Mayo Clinic.[16]

Watch: "Have Type 2 Diabetes? Try Walking After Eating" at **https://www.youtube.com/watch?v=itmdsOUVBcc**

Watch: "Walk for Health: The Best Medicine" at **https://www.youtube.com/watch?v=mbIM1LTfytQ**

Stand Up

Books have been written with titles like "Sitting Kills, Moving Heals: How Everyday Movement Will Prevent Pain, Illness, and Early Death—and Exercise Alone Won't" by Joan Vernikos, Ph.D. or "Get Up!: Why Your Chair is Killing You and What You Can Do About It" by James Levine, MD. Dr. Vernikos was the Director of NASA's Life Sciences from 1993 to 2000, while Dr. Levine has worked for the Mayo Clinic. From the research discussed by both authors, too much sitting can harm health. If we spend up to an hour exercising per day, what do we do the other twenty-three hours? Dr. Joan Vernikos recommends using gravity to our advantage. By just slowly standing up, valuable changes occur in our body—like muscle contractions and nerve stimulations. One benefit of doing this is better blood pressure levels. The process of standing up is the stimulus, not the amount of time standing. The way to get the most benefit from standing up is to do it slowly and **to stand up at least thirty-two times a day.** "Stand up, sit less, move more" summarizes research on avoiding sitting too much.

Standing has its own benefits. For example, Dr. Francisco Lopez-Jimenez's editorial on a research study of "Replacing sitting time with standing or stepping" summarizes the benefits of standing and stepping instead of sitting. The benefits are improved fasting blood glucose and triglyceride levels, and a prevention of atherogenesis (formation of abnormal fatty or lipid masses in arterial walls). Also, standing up and adding some steps will improve weight control.[17] If you work at a desk, research indicates a 20-8-2 ratio for every thirty minutes—sit for twenty minutes, stand for eight, and move for two.[18]

Dr. Joan Vernikos also gives this example of how beneficial standing up can be. Her 99-year-old uncle was hit by a car as he crossed the street. His upper leg bone, the femur, was broken. He was hospitalized. As he was lying in his hospital bed, he called her, asking her what to do. She told him to get out of the hospital as soon as possible, but in the meantime, to sit up every 30 minutes with his legs hanging over the side of the bed, after doing this a couple of minutes to lie back down. Once he was home, she advised him to stand up every 30 minutes. He followed her prescription when he got home, and to the amazement of the orthopedic surgeon, his bone healed in two weeks. So, let's stand up slowly more than thirty-two times daily for health and vitalization.

Strengthen Up

One of the most important factors to know about strength training is the benefits this exercise brings for blood sugar control. The reason is that muscle contractions uptake glucose into the cells of the muscle through another avenue without the use of insulin. Your muscles can continue to bring in more glucose via Glut4 glucose transporters—without insulin initially—for some time after exercise. The muscle stores glucose or glycogen and uses it as an energy source during exercise. When dieting, many people lose not only fat but muscle, too. Think of the muscle as your gas tank or glucose tank that replenishes the expended glycogen supply by uptaking glucose from the blood during and after exercise without insulin and with insulin too. So, it makes your insulin much more effective and sensitive, with less of it needed. In other words, by maintaining muscle mass or increasing the amount of muscle, the body becomes more sensitive to insulin. So, strengthen and build up your muscle mass for better blood sugar control.

When is the best time to do this type of exercise? By doing this after meals, I've discovered I can maintain better blood glucose levels. I am up to eight exercises three times a week with four sets of repetitions for each exercise. I do several exercises for about fifteen minutes after two meals a day. I rotate the exercises of the upper body and lower body muscles every other day. A proper sequence of breathing is essential, too. Breathe out while actually lifting the weight and breathe in while lowering the weight. Don't hold your breath when lifting the weight because high blood pressure can result!

Stretch Out

After you do your strength training exercises, follow them with **stretching exercises** while the muscles are warm, says exercise expert Dr. Sheri Colberg. Some of the benefits she lists are moving and reaching more fully and relaxing stiff, sore, and tired muscles. Also, lowering the risk of sports injuries, preventing falls due to lack of flexibility, and combating the loss of flexibility from aging, inactivity, and diabetes are additional benefits.[19]

Motivation to Exercise

It is amazing what we can do when we have the motivation and see the benefits. Here is an example of someone who overcame insurmountable obstacles and succeeded in training for an Ironman competition. Picture yourself running a 26.2-mile marathon, riding a bicycle 112 miles, and swimming 2.4 miles. Winners in Ironman Triathlon races accomplish all of this in less than fourteen hours. Endurance is needed. No one would doubt Ironman competition is very difficult. It is named "Ironman" not because competitors wear iron suits but because the event is hard, like iron. Ironman Triathlons require willpower. Without training, competing in this competition would be dangerous and ill-advised. We can imagine riding a bicycle around a few blocks in our neighborhood, but who could pedal 112 miles altogether?

This competition is for the young, although there is an instance of 85-year-old Hiromu Inada participating in the race and completing it in 16 hours and 53 minutes. Average winning times are 12 hours and 35 minutes. The willpower of some people is incredible, which brings me to the example of 39-year-old Jay. Not only did he train and compete in this event, but he did so while battling brain cancer. He first saw an Ironman race on TV in 1989 and thought, "they must be superhuman." When his daughter was born, he wanted to show her that she could do unbelievable things, and he would compete when she turned ten. But he started his training early when his daughter was only three. On that day in 2018, when he was diagnosed with brain cancer, he started his training. Last year his finishing time was 13 hours and 40 minutes. This accomplishment came after two brain surgeries, 30 radiation sessions, and a year of chemo.

His performance did not just happen; he had great motivation. During 2020, because of COVID-19, athletes could make their virtual courses. Jay set his finish line in front of his house. When he came around the corner, straining toward the finish line, he could see his home with his wife and daughter (and hundreds of others) cheering him toward the tape. He said, "My daughter and my wife were holding that tape, so I just zeroed in on them, thinking, 'I'm coming home.' I didn't have much energy, but I kissed my wife and got down on my knees to say to my daughter and hero, 'If I can do it, you can do it. Dream big and never give up hope.'" In this scene, we see the motivation that gave him willpower—his family. When it comes to exercising in Wise Way #7, let's focus on the benefits exercise brings for our health and wellness and be motivated by our families, friends, and potential friends we can encourage to practice them![20]

Read this article, "Get Stronger, Live Longer," for descriptions of eight exercises and images of how they are done with neoprene dumbbells.

https://assets.aarp.org/www.aarpmagazine.org_/articles/health/fitness_machines/SmartFitness_FreeWeights.pdf

Stretching exercises are illustrated in this pdf. "Exercises for Older People."

https://www.nhs.uk/Tools/Documents/NHS_ExercisesForOlderPeople.pdf

Inserted 11.8.19 -

https://www.nhs.uk/livewell/fitness/documents/NHS_sitting_exercise.pdf

For a full explanation of the benefits of exercise, read the article "The Science of Exercise" in Diabetes Forecast magazine.

http://www.diabetesforecast.org/2010/jul/the-science-of-exercise.html

CHAPTER TWO

Wise Ways to Stay in Control During the Afternoon

*"She (wisdom) will give you a garland to grace
your head and present you with a glorious crown.
Listen, my son, accept what I say, and the years
of your life will be many"* (Proverbs 4:9-10).

8 Stay Hydrated

*Drink Cold Water—"Like cold water to a weary soul is
good news from a distant land"* (Proverbs 25:25).

Remember, when reading the proverb above, the statement made of God's wisdom teachings in Proverbs 4:22—*"They are life to those who find them and health to one's whole body."* The basic meaning of the word *proverb* is to represent, compare, or be like. Proverbs are pictures of reality. What better way to picture the gratifying, exuberant effect that good news has on a person than with the image of the satisfaction cold water gives a thirsty person? *"Like cold water to a weary soul is good news from a distant land"* (Proverbs 25:25).

Proverbs have more than one dimension, and the meaning here is not just about good news. In other words, the consequence of good news is pictured with the wonderful feeling that cold water gives to a thirsty person. And guess what? Cold water is good for our health.

I recently visited a worker at a supermarket. I overheard her tell a customer how she was feeling with her diabetes. Then, I had a short visit with her. She told me that she drinks water to bring down her blood glucose level, which amazingly works sometimes. Why? Dehydration makes a person feel fatigued. It can also elevate the stress hormone cortisol. Cortisol is a counterregulatory hormone to insulin. Thus, when cortisol levels are elevated, insulin is less effective. The result is elevated blood sugar levels.

Drink Water! *"Like a snow-cooled drink at harvest time is a trustworthy messenger to the one who sends him; he refreshes the spirit of his master."* (Proverbs 25:13). Doctor Willett of Harvard Medical School teaches drinking sixty-four ounces of water a day for a person on a 2,000-calorie meal plan.[21] Others have suggested drinking half an ounce for every pound you weigh and an ounce for every minute you exercise to keep hydrated. French researchers discovered drinking thirty-four ounces of water per day prevented elevated blood glucose in a nine-year study of 3600 individuals.[22] Eating whole foods rich in water also makes a difference in the amount to drink. Most fruits and vegetables are mainly water. Notice the water content in the following foods: fruits and vegetables (80–95%), hot cereal (85%), low-fat fruit-flavored yogurt (75%), boiled egg (75%), and fish and seafood (60–85%). When we compare a popular junk food like potato chips, we discover it has only 2 percent water content.[23]

What about carbonated soft drinks? According to Doctor Willett, these drinks work for staying hydrated but are loaded with sugar. And sugar-free artificially sweetened soda drinks are a concern. Many are wary of artificial sweeteners.[24] If that is a concern, get an Infuser for fruit-infused water!

A way to determine dehydration is the color of urine. For example, the dark yellow or yellowish-brown color could indicate dehydration.[25] "Studies have shown that being just half a liter (about 17 ounces) dehydrated can increase your cortisol levels," says Amanda Carlson, RD, director of performance nutrition at Athletes' Performance—a training clinic for world-class athletes. "Cortisol is one of those stress hormones. Staying in a good hydrated status can keep your stress levels down. When you don't give your body the fluids it needs, you're putting stress on it, and it's going to respond to that," says Amanda Carlson.[26] Dehydration can elevate blood glucose because cortisol levels can increase, causing resistance to insulin. In addition, with fewer bodily fluids, blood decreases, also causing low blood pressure.

Another consideration for weight loss is to drink water. Are you hungry or just need to drink something? Feeling hungry may signal the need for more fluids. How can you distinguish thirst from hunger? Sip a glass of ice water before grabbing something to eat, and then wait five to ten minutes. Thirty-six ounces of cold water daily can elevate metabolism and calorie burning by one hundred calories per day, a study reveals. A benefit of drinking water cold comes when drinking ice cold water. Ice cold water requires energy to warm it to core body temperature.[27]

How many calories will you burn to bring an ice-cold sixteen-ounce drink to body temperature? One calorie is burned for each ounce of iced beverage to warm it to core body temperature. Drinking sixty-four ounces of ice-cold water a day results in burning sixty-four calories.[28]

Staying hydrated and drinking ice-cold water is vital for those with health concerns, which is all of us, isn't it? Wisdom's way teaches, *"The mind of a person with understanding gets knowledge; the wise person listens to learn more"* (Proverbs 18:15 NCV).

I drink small amounts of water throughout the day—six glasses with six to eight ounces of water each time. To drink it all at once isn't good for you! I combine drinking water with eating water-rich foods like vegetables and fruit. *"The wisdom of the prudent is to give thought to their ways"* (Proverbs 14:8).

9 Wisely Eat Healthy Snacks, Nutrition—what about eggs?

Does An Apple a Day Keep the Doctor Away?

"Make plans by seeking advice; if you wage war, obtain guidance" (Proverbs 20:18). We all like snacks, but some snacks are unhealthy, like donut holes. So, to win the war against poor health, we need guidance or advice to make wise choices for snacks. If you follow an intermittent fasting schedule, like 16 hours of fasting and an eight-hour window for eating or 18:6, time will be the first factor for restricting snacks. No snacks

that will break your fast! You can drink black coffee, tea, or water and non-calorie flavoring. I will recommend intermittent fasting in the 14th wise way. Knowledge is knowing a tomato or avocado is a fruit; wisdom is not putting it on a fruit salad. Knowledge is knowing donuts, donut holes, chips, pretzels, and a bucket of buttered popcorn at the theater are snacks; wisdom is replacing them with healthy snacks!

What are the benefits of snacking? Snacking helps prevent overeating at meals, and it provides a constant source of nutritional fuel. The body also gets a regular supply of fuel, which can help prevent low blood glucose levels when using insulin or sulfonylureas like Glipizide, Glimepiride, and Glyburide. Of course, before fasting, consult your doctor if you are on medications like these.

What are some good snacks to eat? I would cautiously eat fresh fruits in small quantities because they stimulate insulin production. So when eating an apple, it should be a small portion like half or a cup or four ounces of cherries, half of a grapefruit, twelve or fewer grapes, and half of an orange, peach, or pear. These are good snacks from the criteria of being low-glycemic. A popular snack is a donut hole, or should we say donut holes! A single donut hole weighs only half an ounce and has fifty-two calories! Whereas 5.1 ounces of strawberries have only forty-six calories! Which one will give you a more-full feeling for a snack? Low-calorie density foods, which add more volume of food to your snack, are also high-density nutrient snacks. One donut hole has sugar, saturated fat, and flour. In contrast, the 5.1-ounce serving of strawberries has virtually no fat but has water and three grams of fiber. When we subtract the fiber, it has only thirty-four calories and anti-inflammatory antioxidants (antioxidants stop or delay damage to the cells). Strawberries have omega 3 and 6 fatty acids, minerals like magnesium, potassium, and calcium, and vitamins like A, C, E, and K. So eat low–glycemic index carbohydrates that don't spike up blood sugars.

Raw vegetables are even better snacks. Eat them with a lower-fat dip or with different flavored mustards. At our Diabetes Support Group, one person told me she's enjoying eating radishes and losing weight. Radishes? Yes, she's eating radishes. Radishes are rich in fiber, vitamin C, and potassium. One cup of raw radishes has only 19 calories and 4 grams of carbohydrates, but 1.7 grams of fiber. Another person said he's been eating mushrooms and has noticed better blood glucose control. Mushrooms have 23 calories for one cup with 2 grams of carbohydrates. They are also anti-inflammatory foods.

Radishes and mushrooms are much better choices than potato chips and pretzels. They are more filling. Radishes are about 90% water. In comparison, potato chips have about 2% water. One serving (28 grams) of chips has 160 calories, 15 grams of carbohydrates, and 10 grams of fat. One serving (28 grams) of pretzels has 100 calories and 23 grams of carbohydrates. Do not eat these for snacks!

Deli meat wrapped in romaine lettuce leaves, low-fat cottage cheese and fruit, a boiled egg, smoked salmon, or tuna with vegetables would all be good options. Remember, the calories add up quickly in nuts like almonds, walnuts, and pecans. Portion control is essential for nuts! Again, the calories add up quickly.

What about eggs? Here are what several doctors say about eggs and their benefits. Dr. Marty Makary in his new book Blind Spots writes, "Study after study has failed to demonstrate the connection between dietary cholesterol and heart disease, or between the cholesterol in your diet and the cholesterol levels in your blood. To the contrary, strong scientific research has revealed a stark reality: The cholesterol you eat is generally not absorbed by the body. That's because the vast majority of cholesterol in food has a bulky side-chain molecule connected to it that does not allow it to be absorbed."[29]

Dr. Ghada Soliman of City University of New York researched in 2018, dozens of studies on this topic and wrote, "Extensive research did not show evidence to support a role of dietary cholesterol in the development of CVD [cardiovascular disease]. Considering that eggs are affordable and nutrient-dense food items, containing high-quality protein...it would be worthwhile to include eggs in moderation as a part of a healthy eating pattern."[30]

In fact, there are several benefits of eggs. First, notice what Dr. Fung writes. "Potential egg nutritional benefits include increased weight loss, better skin and eye health, enhanced liver and brain function and a reduced risk of heart disease and metabolic syndrome. Free-range eggs, in particular, tend to be safer, more ethically produced and higher in several important nutrients. Studies now conclude that eating eggs, even daily, does not raise the risk of heart disease. In fact, consuming lots of eggs reduces the risk of diabetes by 42 percent."[31]

Dr. Eric Berg says this in a Youtube presentation. "Egg protein has the greatest anabolic effect—48% of egg protein is converted into body protein. This means it goes directly into your muscles and joints. Your body is only able to convert 32% of the protein in meat and fish." "Studies have shown that if you consume whole eggs, your body is more efficient at building muscle and you have a shorter recovery time after exercise. The insulin index is a scale that classifies how different non-carbohydrate foods affect insulin. Whole eggs have a much lower effect on insulin than egg whites alone. When you remove the fat from a protein source, you have a greater insulin spike." Dr Berg eats 4 eggs per day. I eat an average of three eggs per day. Do your research and make a wise decision.

Dr. Josh Axe, DNM, DC, CNS, is a certified doctor of natural medicine, doctor of chiropractic, and clinical nutritionist. He lists on his website "51 Healthy Snack Ideas." His ideas with recipes include such snacks as "Baked Cinnamon Apple Chips, Five-Minute Healthy Strawberry Yogurt, Paleo Apple 'Nachos,' Raw Homemade Applesauce, Very Cherry Snack Bar, Cajun Roasted Chickpeas, Zucchini Chips, Crispy Chickpea Bites, Healthy Spicy Black Bean Dip, Healthy Sweet Potato Nachos, Paprika and Chili Kale Chips, Quick Crackers, Creamy Avocado Yogurt Dip, Spiced Nuts, Roasted Pumpkin Seeds, Spicy Buffalo Cauliflower Bites and many more. To read the recipes, go to **https://draxe.com/healthy-snack-ideas/** .

Watch: "Travel Foods & Snacks" at **https://www.youtube.com/watch?v=F0eWaR7gJY4&t=10s**

10 Eat Dinner (lunch), Walk, and Take a POWER NAP.

A good conscience is a soft pillow.
I'm so good at sleeping I can do it with my eyes closed.

Why take a nap? Please give me one good reason. Jesus did! Remember what happened on the Sea of Galilee? *"A furious squall came up, and the waves broke over the boat, so that it was nearly swamped. Jesus was in the stern, **sleeping on a cushion"*** (Mark 4:37-38). When was Jesus sleeping? During a storm, yes, during a storm! We find a wisdom insight on how he could do this in Proverbs 3. ***"Do not let wisdom and understanding out of your sight...****Then you will go on your way in safety, and your foot will not stumble. When you lie down, you will not be afraid; when you lie down, **your sleep will be sweet"*** (Proverbs 3:22-24).

Taking naps has been the habit of many famous people like Albert Einstein and Winston Churchill. Albert Einstein took naps! Your IQ may not be off the charts, but when it comes to naps, you and I can be a genius. Einstein believed in power naps. He would sit in his chair and hold a pencil or a spoon as he dozed off. When he dropped it, he knew his nap time was over. Unlike many daytime nappers, Einstein also got plenty of rest at night, regularly sleeping for at least 10 hours. Winston Churchill said, "Nature has not intended mankind to work from eight in the morning until midnight without that refreshment of blessed oblivion which, even if it only lasts twenty minutes, is sufficient to renew all the vital forces... Don't think you will be doing less work because you sleep during the day. That's a foolish notion held by people who have no imaginations. You will be able to accomplish more. You get two days in one—well, at least one and a half." We could add more than Nature, but wisdom, God's wisdom, would condone taking a nap, as seen in Jesus! Dr. Sara Mednick, in her book "Take a Nap; Change Your Life," gives 20 reasons why we should take a nap. Some of the reasons relate to diabetes self-management. The Ninth reason she gives is that sleepy people are more susceptible to junk food cravings. The eleventh reason is to reduce your risk of diabetes or better manage it. Studies reveal sleep deprivation increases cortisol levels. Cortisol, the stress hormone, causes a need for more insulin. Increased levels of cortisol bring resistance to insulin, which then has a direct effect on blood glucose management.[32]

Dr. Mednick reports that sleeplessness causes hypertension, but during sleep, blood pressure decreases. So, when you remain awake longer than normal, your blood pressure can stay higher. This can also result in a higher risk for strokes. In addition, when we deprive ourselves of sleep, we enter a period of overdrive and need extra energy to support physical functions. Also, irritability, anger, depression, and mental exhaustion can be linked with sleeplessness. Dr. Mednick gives these guidelines for napping: keep the room as dark as possible, go for quietness, and stay warm.

"I usually take a two-hour nap from one to four," said Yogi Berra. What is the optimal length of time for a nap? Various lengths of a nap bring different beneficial results. If you have time to nap as long as Yogi, you will sleep through all the stages of sleep. If you don't have that kind of time, even

a twenty-minute nap brings benefits. Those twenty minutes help with rejuvenated alertness and improve motor skills like typing. Thirty to sixty-minute naps or slow-wave sleep brings better decision-making and short-term memory but grogginess when waking. So, during a twenty-minute power nap in the lighter stages of sleep, increased energy and alertness come when awakening. Avoid taking caffeine for up to four hours before you expect to take your nap, and then your nap will become your energy drink!

According to a recent study, one way to remedy the negative effects of a poor night's sleep is to take a short nap the following day.[33] Researchers have found naps to reduce stress and bolster the immune system. The Mayo Clinic lists the following benefits of taking naps: relaxation, reduced fatigue, increased alertness, improved mood and performance, including quicker reaction time and better memory.[34] So, take a nap as your energy drink!

11 Eat Carbs Last as You Slowly Eat— fiber and chia seeds.

Precious Present

"It is not good to have zeal without knowledge, nor to be hasty and miss the way" (Proverbs 19:2).

Someone says, "I've always enjoyed my food. I may eat fast, but it's often because...Well, actually, I've never thought about why I eat fast, but it doesn't really matter, does it?" *"Whoever is patient has great understanding"* (Proverbs 14:29). The following is an example of how patiently eating brings about great understanding for wise mindful eating.

How do we eat? The table is set and ready for food. Twelve hungry brothers sit at the table ready to eat. Mom brings the food and sets it before them. The food is limited and these guys are famished. Can you picture the scene? The only thing you hear is the chomping of teeth. How long will it take for them to clean their plates? I can imagine asking for dessert in five minutes. When you sit down to eat, you're not sitting with eleven hungry brothers are you? Yet, it is so easy to fall into the trap of devouring food without even tasting it.

Imagine a tiger chasing you. Running for your life a sharp deep cliff confronts you. You have no place to go. The tiger is getting so close you can feel him breathing down your neck, then you notice a rope dangling over the cliff and grab it. Holding onto the rope for your life, you sway, dangling from the cliff. The tiger roars above and five hundred feet below sharp jagged rocks invite you to fall. Then you notice two mice chewing on the rope above you. What should you do?

The tiger above, the rocks below and the rope is about to break! Just then you notice delicious-looking bright red, ripe strawberries growing out of the side of the cliff. You stretch out one hand, pluck a strawberry, and pop it into your mouth. The strawberry is so sweet and refreshing. You think "Delicious—that's the best strawberry I've ever tasted."

If you were still occupied with the tiger above or the sharp rocks below, you would have never tasted and enjoyed the strawberries. We call this the *precious present*! When we eat, are we focusing on the smell, texture, color, and rich taste of the food we're eating? Research indicates for most people, the feeling of satiety (fullness) takes about twenty minutes. We haven't given ourselves time for that feeling to catch up because we're gulping down our food!

Sleep Deprivation

Physical health is also impacted by sleep deprivation. There is an impairment of hormones that relate to appetite. Less leptin, the "feel full" hormone is released, and more of ghrelin, the "still hungry" hormone. This makes losing weight an even greater challenge. So, the strategy is to sleep more and lose weight. Adequate sleep relates to the feeling of satiety and to this strategy of eating slowly. Synergy is needed when these two principles of sleep and satiety come together and give you greater results than expected.

Eating Sequence: Eat Carbs Last

So, what can we do? Previous studies have found that eating quickly results in eating more! Eating too fast outpaces the satiety signal (feeling full sensation), which takes about 20 minutes. Could "postprandial" (after meal) blood sugar levels be affected by how fast you eat carbs? Yes, especially if you eat the carbs on your plate first. What is the timing sequence of eating protein and carbs? Eat protein first! What difference does that make? "You've got to be kidding?" God's wisdom instructs us to be mindful of sequence. For example, *"Finish your outdoor work and get your fields ready; after that, build your house"* (Proverbs 24:27). "Carbohydrates raise blood sugar, but if you tell someone not to eat them—or to cut back drastically—it's hard for them to comply," says Dr. Louis Aronne. Researchers at Cornell say, "This study points to an easier way that patients might lower their blood sugar and insulin levels." The research focused on how much and when carbohydrates are eaten. Eleven Type 2 Diabetics who were obese and only on metformin were the research group. Their meals consisted of carbohydrates, protein, vegetables, and fat. They ate carbs first and then waited fifteen minutes to eat protein. Then, they reversed the order. Their blood sugars were checked post-meal every 30, 60, and 120-minute intervals. Eating carbs last brought much better results with 30, 60, and 120-minute checks—by about 29 percent, 37 percent, and 17 percent, respectively.

The Importance of Eating Fiber

A curious factor is shown when we look at food labels. Under the total number of carbohydrates listed, fiber is included. Fiber is a carbohydrate that the body cannot break down, and it has several benefits. Eating foods with fiber means you eat fewer calories, which is also helpful for controlling weight. The book "Glucose Revolution" lists these three superpowers of fiber: First, it reduces the action of an enzyme that breaks starch down into glucose molecules. Second, it slows down stomach emptying: when fiber is present, food moves more slowly. Finally, it creates a dense mesh in the small intestine, making it harder for glucose to reach the bloodstream. Through these designs, fiber slows down the breakdown and absorption of any glucose that lands in the stomach after it. This results in flattening the spike up of glucose. And let me add that this is especially true of soluble fiber, which dissolves in water, becomes a gummy gel, and helps blunt elevated blood glucose after a meal. So fiber (soluble) limits rapid BG peaks, gives a full feeling longer, and helps control cholesterol. A man's goal is to eat 38 grams of fiber per day, and a woman should eat 25 grams per day.

Another way of putting these benefits from the book Glucose Revolution is this. "Fiber is also good for our glucose levels for several reasons, notably because it creates a dense mesh in our intestine. The mesh slows down and reduces the absorption of molecules from food across the intestinal lining. What does this mean for our glucose curves? First, that we absorb fewer calories. And second, with fiber in our system, any absorption of glucose or fructose molecules is lessened."[35]

"Better to have a dish of vegetables where there is love than juicy steaks where there is hate" (Proverbs 15:17). Most people find a delicious steak meal satisfying to the taste, but the taste is lost when eating the meal with bitter, resentful, and hateful people toward you. Whereas eating a meal with those you love is pictured with vegetables. And guess what? As we've been examining, vegetables are good for us. Isn't it interesting that a subtle message of a meal of vegetables shows love? And what are vegetables? They are very beneficial for health. Here are some examples of fruits and vegetables rich in soluble fiber. Start your meals with greens. Any vegetable qualifies, from roasted asparagus to coleslaw to grilled zucchini and grated carrots. We're talking artichokes, broccoli, turnips, brussels sprouts, eggplant, lettuce, tomatoes, and also beans.

Broccoli

Dr. Josh Axe website says this about broccoli. "Broccoli was first cultivated as an edible crop in the northern Mediterranean region starting in about the sixth century B.C. As far back as the Roman Empire, it's been considered a uniquely valuable food when it comes to promoting health and longevity. Believe it or not, it didn't actually become widely known in the U.S. until the 1920s, which is surprising if you consider how popular it is today. Why is broccoli good for dieters? It's one of the most nutrient-dense foods on Earth. One cup of the cooked veggie has just over 50 calories but a good dose of fiber (2.3 grams), protein and detoxifying phytochemicals (which reduce inflammation). Is broccoli a carb? As a complex carbohydrate high in fiber, it is a great choice for supporting balanced blood sugar levels, ongoing energy and helping you feel full. Want to know a secret to losing weight fast? Including more high-volume, low-calorie, high-nutrient foods in your meals is key. Broccoli nutrition is high in volume due to having a high water content, so it takes up room in your stomach and squashes cravings or over-eating without adding lots of calories to meals."[36]

Start Drinking Miracle Water

How can you keep from having glucose spikes after a meal? Eat more fiber or drink it. One of the easiest, most beneficial ways to get more fiber is to drink it with what some call "miracle water." What is that? It is water that includes chia seeds. I first put three tablespoons of chia in a mid-sized glass and then add the water. The seeds absorb the water and expand twelve-fold after about fifteen to twenty minutes. It becomes a thick, nutritious drink with about eight grams of mainly soluble fiber. The result is better blood glucose control. This happens because I begin drinking this "miracle water" before I start eating food at a meal. I do this twice a day, which gives me sixteen grams of primarily soluble fiber. Twenty-five grams and thirty-eight grams are recommended daily for women and men.

Another great benefit I've discovered is consistently healthy bowel movements. If you have problems with constipation or loose bowel movements, start drinking this chia miracle water. These seeds are also rich in omega-3 fatty acids which are a type of polyunsaturated fat and antioxidants like selenium, which fight free radicals that can damage your cells.

Omega-3 fatty acids are beneficial to our health in several ways. These fatty acids can even reduce the metabolic syndrome directly related to diabetes. The symptoms are high amounts of visceral fat, high blood sugar, triglycerides, high blood pressure, and low HDL cholesterol, the good cholesterol. Another good factor they reduce is inflammation. Scientific research also indicates that Omega-3s can help calcium to be absorbed, which affects the issue of osteoporosis. Lowering swelling and inflammation helps people with tender joints and arthritis. They improve exercise performance. Also, reasonable amounts of omega-3 lower the risk of macular degeneration, the leading cause of blindness in people over sixty years old.[37] There are four categories of omega-3 fatty acids—ALA, APA, EPA, and DHA. How can we get more? This is where the wisdom principle of being thoughtful comes into play. *"The wisdom of the prudent is to give thought to their ways, but the folly of fools is deception"* (Proverbs 14:8).

Eating fish is the easiest way to get more of these fatty acids. The ALA comes from plants; you must eat more to absorb more. One gram is in a 3.5-ounce serving of albacore (white) tuna. Salmon is another good source with DHA (1.24 grams) and EPA (0.59 grams). ALA has 2.53 grams in a tablespoon of chia seeds.[38] So, make it a lifestyle point to consume more omega-3s.

Soluble Fiber

Here is a contrast between high soluble fiber raw vegetables like bell peppers and carrots which have very little impact on blood sugar levels compared to dry cereal like Rice Krispies. I did a check on my blood sugar and discovered that just twenty-three grams of Rice Krispies with four grams of milk almost doubled my blood sugar level from 100 mg/dl to 175 mg/dl in less than forty minutes.

In contrast to dry cereal, beans are loaded with fiber and especially soluble fiber. The following list gives serving size, total fiber grams per serving, and the number of soluble fiber grams in each serving. Black beans ½ cup 6.1, 2.4 Kidney beans, light red ½ cup 7.9, 2.0 Lima beans ½ cup 4.3, 1.1 Navy beans ½ cup 6.5, 2.2 Pinto beans ½ cup 6.1, 1.4. The best options to keep your glucose levels steady are berries—Strawberries 1 ¼ cup 2.8 (1.1), citrus fruits—oranges 1 small 2.9 (1.8), and apples—with skin 1 small 2.8 (1.0) because they contain the most fiber and the smallest amount of sugar. The worst options—because they have the highest amount of sugar—are mangoes, pineapple, and other tropical fruit. Make sure you eat something else before you eat the fruit. Eat fruit last. It makes a good dessert.

Eating Whole Foods

Eating healthy is a challenge, especially when there are so many delicious unhealthy temptations. People think that if they practice some portion control, they will succeed. Like Yogi Berra said, "When the waitress asked if I wanted my pizza cut into four or eight slices, I said, 'Four. I don't think I can eat eight." People use fad diets to shed pounds quickly. But, unfortunately, once the weight is lost, the old habits return, and so do the pounds and then some. Dr. Jennifer Hubert of St. Joseph Health Medical Group calls this yo-yo dieting. Dr. Hubert says, "Other findings indicate that yo-yo dieting may lead to a higher risk of increased body fat, which means these diets, in the long run, can have the opposite of the intended effect of losing weight. What's worse is that most yo-yo dieting is done with the trendy diets of the moment, which are poor nutritionally compared to eating a regular diet of whole foods like this video is showing."[39]

Whole foods are like the difference between an apple and apple juice. The way to have fruit is in its whole state, with all the nutrients still there. Plus, in the whole state, foods are much more filling! Healthy whole foods are naturally loaded with fiber, vitamins, and minerals. Some are antioxidants that protect cells against damage. Whole foods are rich, nutrient-dense foods. They have no added sugars and fats and exclude added salt or other high-sodium ingredients.

Three More Ways to Disarm the Effects of Carbs on Blood Glucose

When my wife and I were on a trip recently, we went to eat at a restaurant. Before leaving my hotel room, I ate some nuts.

Once there, I ordered some thick bacon, scrambled eggs with a variety bowl of fruits, and a biscuit. Once the waitress brought the food, I ate my bacon and eggs first and then cut my biscuit in half and ate it with some of the fruit. After eating, I took a fifteen-minute walk back to the hotel. My blood sugar stayed within 100 to 140 mg/dl.

Why am I telling you this? Since carbohydrates directly affect blood glucose levels, use fat to blunt or disarm their effects. Fifteen minutes before you eat your meal, eat some cheese and nuts. And here is Why? Fat will affect the pyloric sphincter, a valve from the stomach to the small intestine. The fat causes it to begin to tighten, which causes the absorption of carbohydrates to slow and helps prevent a glucose spike. The pyloric valve is a muscular ring that regulates the speed by which food leaves the stomach and goes into the intestine.

Dr. Rob Thompson writes, "As soon as fat passes through your pyloric valve and reaches your intestine, it activates a reflex that closes the pyloric valve, which keeps food from exiting the stomach. It doesn't take much fat to do this. Scientists have found that as little as two teaspoons (10 g) of fat before a meal will slow stomach emptying. If you eat a fatty snack— a piece of cheese or a handful of nuts— 10 or 15 minutes before a meal, it will close the pyloric valve. When you sit down to eat, you will still have plenty of room in your stomach to enjoy your meal. However, because the tightened pyloric valve slows the passage of food out of your stomach, it takes less food to fill you up. You'll ultimately end up eating less."[40] So eat some cheese and nuts fifteen minutes before a meal for this to happen.

Another thing I did on this trip at another meal was to eat a bowl of salad with vinaigrette dressing first. I've discovered an effortless thing you can do is eat or drink vinegar. Why? Because it slows down the process of breaking down the complex carbohydrates into glucose. The enzyme that does this is amylase. Dr Rob Thompson writes this. "Vinegar inhibits amylase and has been proven to slow the absorption of starch in humans. It has been used for centuries to treat Diabetes. Studies show that 2 tablespoons (30 ml) consumed before eating starch lowers the after-meal glucose and reduces demands for insulin. Vinegar doesn't have to be consumed straight. It can be sprinkled on food as a condiment— a common practice in Mediterranean countries— or used in a salad dressing."[41]

The third thing I did on my trip to disarm the glucose spike effect of carbohydrates was walk after eating, not nap. Do that after you walk. The time of walking is essential. When you walk for a few minutes, your body becomes more sensitive to insulin for the time you are walking and up to the following 48 hours. Plus, your body uses two avenues to reduce blood glucose levels after eating. Insulin is one avenue, and the glucose tranporter—Glut4. As I mentioned in # 7, research indicates you can potentially reduce by half how high your blood glucose will elevate. So do these three things to help control blood glucose: eat cheese and nuts fifteen minutes before eating, eat a salad with some vinegar dressing, and take a short walk after eating.

Walk With the Wise Like Thomas Edison

If you can't seem to eliminate junk food, then don't give up. Instead, look to those who didn't give up even under very trying situations, like Thomas Edison! Edison described himself as deaf, but in fact, he was not totally deaf. It is more accurate to say he was very hard of hearing. He once wrote, "I have not heard a bird sing since I was twelve years old." So, why didn't Edison invent a hearing aid? He often told reporters that he was working on one; sometimes, he tested hearing aids designed by others. But it seems that Edison saw advantages to being deaf. For example, he said that it helped him concentrate on his work. In 1927, he told a group of 300 hard-of-hearing adults, "Deaf people [like himself] should take to reading. It beats the babble of ordinary conversation." Thomas Edison's labs burned in 1914. He said, "Our greatest weakness lies in giving up. The most certain way to succeed is always to try just one more time." The way of wisdom states that *"A wise man has great power and a man of knowledge increases strength"* (Proverbs 24:5). The best way to do "one more time" is with more knowledge.

105-Year-Old Ida Keeling

The following story tells of a woman winning a race at one hundred-five years old. When I read her story, I was impressed with her insights about living. Ida Keeling won and broke the world record for her age group—100 years old at the 122nd Penn Relays. Ida didn't start running until she was sixty-seven! A family tragedy of the murder of her two sons motivated her daughter, Shelly Keeling, to enroll her in a 5K run. "She was just sitting at home in gloom. I just picked her up one morning and said, 'You're coming with me,' and I bought her an extra pair of sneakers, and the rest is history." What is her secret to longevity? "Eat for nutrition, not for taste," she said. "Do what you need to do, not what you want to do, and make sure you exercise at least once every day." And as an afterthought in the story, She said, "I thank God every day for my blessings." And why not![42]

Guidelines Summary of Eating Slowly and Eating Carbs Last

The Joslin Diabetes Center has a program called "Why WAIT? Weight Achievement and Intensive Treatment for Diabetes." Mindful eating is taught.[43] Take your time. Don't get in a big hurry in eating. They suggest relaxing and taking a couple of minutes of deep breathing. Look at the food, noticing its color and texture. (Pretend you will get a grade on a 200-word description you will write of the food!) Smell the food, inhaling the aroma before taking your first bite. Serve yourself less food than you think you need. Taste and savor every bite, chewing it thoroughly. To slow down your pace of eating, put down your fork between each bite. Before deciding to go back for seconds, wait twenty minutes.

And follow these ideas. Take a sip of water between bites. If eating with others, pace yourself with the slow eater. Avoid the "just one more helping" request. Leave some food on your plate. Pre-regulate consumption by deciding how much to eat prior to the meal.

Watch: "Why WAIT? Weight Achievement and Intensive Treatment for Diabetes" at **https://www.youtube.com/ watch?v=9r_Aw70TZGE**

Watch: "Love to Eat? How to Eat and NOT Gain Weight" **https://www.youtube.com/watch?v=cF_zd1LxkuE**

CHAPTER THREE

Wise Ways to Stay in Control During the Evening

"I instruct you in the way of wisdom and lead you along straight paths. When you walk, your steps will not be hampered; when you run, you will not stumble. Hold on to instruction, do not let it go; guard it well, for it is your life" (Proverbs 4:11-13).

12 Use Tools Throughout the Day— Fitness Trackers, (weight loss medications, but with major side effects), balance etc.

Yogi Berra on travel gear: "Why buy good luggage, you only use it when you travel."

For the best blood glucose management results, use tools. Proverbs 14:4 states, *"Where there are no oxen, the feed box is empty. But a strong ox brings in a great harvest."* In ancient times, oxen were essential farming equipment (compare Deuteronomy 22:1, 10). Remember these proverbs are *"life to those who find them and health to one's whole body"* (Proverbs

4:22). The application is not oxen for our health, but tools like food scales, measuring cups, food labels, smaller plates, walking shoes that give comfort and support, a clock for timing of meds, meals, and pedometers or fitness trackers for movement and sleep, record booklets or health apps and glucose meters or continuous glucose monitor systems like the FreeStyle Libre, Medtronic Guardian 4, or Dexcom g7. So, good tools will equip us for better health.

One of the best tools for counting carbs in whole foods is the EatSmartTM Digital Nutrition Scale, which calculates carbs, fiber, and fats. There is a database with nutritional values for a thousand foods. For example, the number of apples is 002. After removing the core and placing the apple on the scale, the scale will show the total calories with grams of carbohydrates and fiber.

> **Watch:** EatSmartTM Digital Nutrition Scale "Weight Loss Tool—Count Calories—EatSmart Nutrition Scale" at https://www.youtube.com/watch?v=AbM4Fbf9OPU

A pedometer or fitness tracker is one of the best motivational tools for getting more steps each day. Researchers conducted a study with two groups wearing pedometers. The participants in one group wore a pedometer with a goal of 10,000 steps daily. The other group's goal was to take a brisk, thirty-minute walk daily. The pedometers worn by the brisk, thirty-minute-a-day walking group were non-viewable. The group using the viewable pedometers averaged over 10,000 steps per day. In comparison, the thirty-minute walking group only walked an average of 8,270 steps—a difference of almost a mile per day.

The following are comments from participants in the 2001 Diabetes in Control 10,000-step research study on the benefits of using a pedometer: "I reduced my stress levels." "It was very easy to just put on the pedometer and check it during the day—it really works." "I never thought I could get to ten thousand steps a day, but just by tracking my steps and increasing ten percent a week, I was able to do it!" "I was surprised to see that it became a habit after just a short time." "My whole family wanted pedometers, and they also increased their steps." "Just by removing the remote controllers, we picked up four hundred steps." "My dog is healthier than ever (I wore the pedometer, not the dog)." "I have more energy, and my blood sugars have never been better. Now my doctor is wearing a pedometer." "My blood pressure is down to normal." "My clothes all fit better." The following are more beneficial tools to use.

Plate Size: "Brian Wansink, Mindless Eating" Interview concerning plate size and how the size helps with portion control at **https://www.youtube.com/watch?v=mP5AFkWZ3eY**

How much movie theater popcorn do people eat? Does it depend on how hungry they are or how good it tastes? Could the size of the box influence how much one eats? Dr. Wansink did a study to determine the influence of the box size on the amount eaten. At a theater in Chicago at a 1:05 p.m. showing, people were given a free box of popcorn. Researchers gave some of them a large box and others a medium-sized box.

They asked participants to answer a few concession stand questions after the movie. They were also to return their bucket or box with any uneaten popcorn. The only catch was they didn't tell the participants the popcorn was five days old.

They did keep it in sterile conditions. Participants were told, "We have found that the average person who is given a large-size container eats more than if they are given a medium-size container. Do you think you ate more because you had the large size?" Most of the participants disagreed. They thought the container size did not affect the amount one would eat. The big-bucket group ate 173 more calories than the medium-sized group. They ate 53 percent more than those with medium-sized boxes. The conclusion was that people eat more when given a bigger container!

What would be a good application for using that information on a daily basis? For example, if you spoon four ounces of sweet potatoes onto a twelve-inch plate, it will look much less than if you had spooned it onto an eight-inch plate. Why not put your food on a midsize plate instead of a larger plate, giving it the appearance of holding more food? We all need to restrict the amount of food we eat to the proper portion size. This could be an easy strategy to use to aid with that goal. The way of wisdom says, *"The wise in heart are called discerning"* (Proverbs 16:21).

- Calorie-free salad dressings: Walden Farms no calorie dressings—**https://www.waldenfarms.com/**
- Shoes: Go-Walk Skechers Shoes
- Pedometers and Fitness Trackers (They monitor different actions like tracking daily steps and measuring heart rate and sleep quality. My family uses the Fitbit Charge 2, 5, or Inspire.)
- Introducing Fitbit Charge 5 In-Depth Review **https://**

www.youtube.com/watch?v=c7KHBR-xSlc
- Labels: "Label Reading 101" at https://www.youtube.com/watch?v=MrdCBqFYDyo

Always when looking at labels, count the carbs. Since the body does not metabolize the fiber, subtract the amount. Doing this is very important for those with ratios to determine how much insulin to give to cover the carbs eaten. The greater the saturated fat, the longer the body metabolizes the carbohydrates. If you use an insulin pump, use the dual mode to extend the amount of time the insulin is delivered. When you see sugar alcohol on the label, you should calculate half the amount for insulin ratios because half is metabolized and affects blood glucose levels.

If you were instructed to keep good records of your blood sugar readings, the amount of food you eat each day, and the number of steps you take each day, would you say, "You've got to be kidding"? Or "I've never done such a silly thing"? However, the way of wisdom states the concept with this principle: *"Be sure you know the condition of your flocks, give careful attention to your herds"* (Proverbs 27:23). Most of us do not have flocks, but we each have a body, and we need to keep track of a herd of health issues like the condition of our blood glucose levels, blood pressure, amount and quality of sleep, exercise and movement and foods. In other words, we need to keep a daily personal health inventory. One way to do this is to keep a food diary along with records of blood glucose readings. Mynetdiary or Fitbit are two of many apps available. Using a tool like this helps with weight loss. In the *Journal of the American Dietetic Association*, an article titled "Food Records: A Predictor and Modifier of Weight Change in a Long-Term Weight Loss Program" concluded: "Those who most accurately recorded their food consumption lost the most weight."

Mynetdiary App. Watch: "MyNetDiary Overview" **https:// www.youtube.com/watch?v=gVAjjkPsAY4**

Ozempic and Mounjaro

Research studies prove Ozempic (semaglutide) causes weight loss. One study showed that participants in a trial lost 10-15% of their body weight over a little more than a year with weekly Ozempic injections combined with healthy eating and exercise. Only 2% of people in the placebo group lost weight, but in the Ozempic group, about 75% lost 5% or more of their body weight. There is another innovative medication called Mounjaro, whose result for weight loss for 84 weeks was 26.6%.

Ozempic and Mounjaro are new medications that have brought outstanding results for people with Type 2 diabetes, including losing weight. People inject these medications once-a-week and do much better with blood sugar control. They also have suppressed hunger, resulting in tremendous weight loss. What do these medications do? They increase insulin sensitivity while inhibiting the liver from releasing glucagon to help lower blood sugar levels. They also suppress appetite and slow digestion, causing many people to lose weight. Due to its long duration of action, people take it once weekly, making it convenient.

These are two among many GLP-1 agonists. They increase the effectiveness of this incretin hormone messenger for insulin production. After you eat, cells in your intestines release GLP-1. They trigger insulin release and block glucose release from the liver. They also slow down how fast food leaves your stomach, making you feel full. GLP-1 is also thought to directly affect the appetite control area of your brain, as well as certain hunger hormones.[44] The GLP-1 can act on brain neuronal circuits in the hypothalamus involved in appetite control. The difference between the medications is that Mounjaro (tirzepatide) is a dual GLP-1/GIP receptor agonist. This means it increases the activity of gut peptides that promote satiety, while GIP also stimulates lipolysis—the breakdown of fat for energy use. Dr. Beverly Tchang says, "We think tirzepatide's weight loss effect is driven more by the GIP component than the GLP-1 effects, and this may be the reason why we are seeing more weight loss from tirzepatide than with other medications, which are only GLP-1 agonists."[45]

Side Effects of Weight Loss Medication

This proverb applies. *"The wisdom of the prudent is to give thought to their ways, but the folly of fools is deception"* (Proverbs 14:8). Here are some of the side effects that people more commonly experience from these weight loss medications. They are nausea, vomiting, constipation, abdominal pain, cramping, and diarrhea. The good news is they only last a short time while beginning the medications.

A longer-term side effect is "Ozempic Face." "The most prominent feature of 'Ozempic face' is the loss of facial fat, which gives a hollowed appearance to the face," explains Dr. Hosseinipour. "This includes a more sunken appearance of the eyes and more prominent jowls, [which is] sagging, loose skin of the jawline."[46] Also, these medications can affect not only the loss of fat but muscle mass as well. What if you can't afford this expensive medication or decide you've lost enough weight and decide to stop using it? "Ozempic Rebound," where people regain most of the weight lost because they don't have lifestyle changes.[47]

Muscle Mass Loss

Here is the most important side effect to consider before beginning one of these medications—muscle mass loss. It is true that people can lose up to sixty-one percent fat, but the other factor is the loss of thirty-nine percent muscle.[48] Why is this so important? Let me explain it with Proverbs 24:5— *"A wise man is strong; and a man of knowledge makes strength greater."*

I put off strength training for years, especially since I walked more than 10,000 steps daily. You don't even have to go to the gym for strength training. Instead, in your home, use neoprene dumbbells that you hold in each hand. If you don't see the value in this training, consider this proverb. *"A wise man is strong; and a man of knowledge makes strength greater"* (Proverbs 24:5). The proverb does mention strong and strength, but isn't that just talking about being resiliently strong in stressful situations, enduring or bouncing back from setbacks in life? Yes, but remember what the purpose of these proverbs is. *"Do not let them out of your sight, keep them within your heart; for they are life to those who find them and health to one's whole body"* (Proverbs 4:21-22). They include health for one's whole body. A person who has more knowledge can also have greater physical strength.

Another proverb says, *"If you falter in a time of trouble, how small is your strength!"* (Proverbs 24:10) If you're going to endure difficult situations, you must work on your attitude and bodily strength. The older we get, the more dangerous falling is to our health and wellness. So I see the proverb applying to physical strength as well as mental. The reason is what is known as sarcopenia, muscle loss with aging. Most men lose 30% of their muscle mass during a lifetime. Consider the results with the wasting away of muscle. There is a 2.3 times greater risk of having a fracture from a fall, such as a broken hip, collarbone, leg, arm, or wrist from sarcopenia. One-third of people aged sixty-five and older fall once a year and a half are in their eighties. The results can be debilitating bone fractures. That describes what could happen with less muscle mass. I've already mentioned research indicates a loss of 39% muscle mass loss with these mediations. Dr Mark Hyman explains "Here's the rub: you have to take it (Ozempic) forever, it's expensive, and most people are not aware that not only do you lose fat but you lose muscle. Nobody is talking about the bad side and, by the way, they're thinking of giving it to five-year-old kids which is just terrifying to me."

Balance

Imagine two different lifestyles as one ages. One path pictures a person rarely walking, working at a desk job before a computer, and then relaxing at home in a recliner watching TV using a remote control. As this person ages, he becomes weaker and weaker. When walking, the person now needs a walker, and then with fewer muscles, a wheelchair is required, and finally, a powered wheelchair. Then comes a bedfast scene before death.

The other path has an active, lively, energetic person walking, jogging, hiking with a backpack, and lifting weights. This is the path of a high-quality, vibrant, vigorous lifestyle. The good news is that older people can reverse muscle loss by doing resistance exercises.[49] By choosing a resistance exercise path, a person can have a spry, active, stable, and healthy lifestyle! Let's decide on that path! I am.

Where are you in this aging process? The Mayo Clinic wrote the results of a recent research study that will help us determine where we are in the aging process and what we can do about it.[50] Answer this question. Can you stand on one leg at a time for thirty seconds? What will that tell you, if you can? Research at the Mayo Clinic had forty participants over fifty, half of whom were 65 to 83. They had them do several things for their study, but standing on one foot at a time was the most critical factor. "Balance is an important measure because, in addition to muscle strength, it requires input from vision, the vestibular system (vestibular sense, also known as the movement, gravity and/or balance sense, allows us to move smoothly and comes from the inner ear.) and the somatosensory systems (somatic neurons enable movement, and the ability to feel the sensations of touch, vibration, pressure, heat and cold.)," says Kenton Kaufman, Ph.D. He also writes, "Changes in balance are noteworthy. If you have poor balance, you're at risk of falling, whether or not you're moving. Falls are a severe health risk with serious consequences."[51]

Their research indicates the highest rate of age decline if you can't stand for thirty seconds, especially on the non-dominant leg. This test is a simple yet effective way to assess your balance and strength. "If you can't stand on your leg for five seconds, you're at risk of falls. If a person can stand on their leg for 30 seconds, they're doing really well, especially if they're older," says Dr. Kaufman.[52] So, it is not hopeless if you can't stand for thirty seconds on one leg. You can practice standing on one leg and improve your balance. Dr. Kaufman says, "If you don't use it, you lose it. If you use it, you maintain it. It's easy to do. It doesn't require special equipment, and you can do it every day."[53]

But here is the problem with Ozempic, Wegovy, Mounjaro, and Zepbound—loss of muscle mass. Should they be taken as a quick fix to lose weight? Johann Hari in his book Magic Pill writes, "Heath Schmidt, the head of the Lab of Neuropsychopharmacology at Penn State University, told me: 'You're not just losing fat when you're on these drugs. Some individuals are also losing 20 to 30 percent lean [muscle] mass, which in the long term could be problematic.'"[54] Many people will benefit from these medications if they make lifestyle changes. To prevent loss of muscle mass, you must practice resistance exercises (Wise Way # 7), increase your protein intake (Wise Way # 5), eat high-nutrition foods that contain an abundance of minerals and vitamins (Wise Ways # 9 and # 11), and stay hydrated (Wise Way # 8).[55] **A way to remedy this weight loss method with these medications is to instead use the discipline of intermittent fasting. For more information on this wise way, read Wise Way # 14.**

13 Eat supper (dinner) earlier with less saturated fat and carbs.

"Eat Breakfast Like a King, Lunch Like a Prince, and Dinner Like a Pauper"

Wisdom's way teaches the following on the importance of timing: *"Anyone who refuses to work doesn't plow in the right season. When he looks for a crop at harvest time, he doesn't find it"* (Proverbs 20:4 NIrV). *"Finish your outdoor work. Get your fields ready. After that, build your house"* (Proverbs 24:27). *"A person finds joy in giving an apt reply—and how good is a timely word!"* (Proverbs 15:23). *"It is not good to have zeal without knowledge, nor to be hasty and miss the way"* (Proverbs 19:2).

Researchers in Spain studied 420 participants in a 20-week weight-loss treatment program.[56] The research answered, "Could the timing of when you eat, be just as important as what you eat?" The meal with the most calories was the lunch meal. They ate forty percent of their daily calories at lunch. The timing of when to eat was the factor analyzed to determine if the time made a difference in weight loss. Researchers divided participants into two groups—early eaters and late eaters. The early eaters ate their lunch before 3 p.m., and the late eaters any time after 3 p.m.

Those who lost significantly less weight and at a slower rate were in the late eaters group. In that group, they ate fewer calories for breakfast and often skipped breakfast. Insulin resistance also increased. But instead, eat breakfast like a king, but be sure to cut back on carbohydrates. Ideally, eating fifteen grams of carbohydrates along with plenty of eggs will help you maintain better blood glucose levels. "Our results indicate that late eaters displayed a slower weight-loss rate and lost significantly less weight than early eaters, suggesting that the timing of large meals could be an important factor in a weight loss program," said Frank Scheer, Ph.D., assistant professor of medicine at Harvard Medical School, and senior author on this study. Not only will eating late make it easier to gain weight, but it also makes it more challenging to maintain blood sugar control. So, the lesson is to try to eat the evening meal early. The amounts of fat and carbohydrates will also determine your blood glucose management.

Someone says, "Your blood glucose is affected by sugar and carbs, so avoid them. Don't worry about other types of food!" However, wisdom's way says, *"The mind of a person with understanding gets knowledge; the wise person listens to learn more"* (Proverbs 18:15 NCV). Is fatty food just the shy, harmless guy sitting in the back row? When you eat fatty foods, they have a powerful metabolic punch. Free fatty acids (FFAs) in the blood increase with high–saturated fat meals. What does that do? Insulin resistance increases with high–saturated fat meals with carbohydrates. With that resistance, you need more insulin to break through the insulin resistance barrier. This compounds blood glucose control for those with Type 1 diabetes and many with Type 2 diabetes with high insulin resistance. A Researcher wrote, "Current guidelines for intensive treatment of type 1 diabetes base the mealtime insulin bolus calculation exclusively on carbohydrate counting. There is strong evidence that free fatty acids impair insulin sensitivity. We hypothesized that patients with type 1 diabetes would require more insulin coverage for higher-fat meals than lower-fat meals with identical carbohydrate content."[57]

High-Fat Dinners vs. Low-Fat Dinners

This study had two meal plans: a High-fat dinner and a Low-Fat dinner. Seven people with Type 1 diabetes participated. They took additional insulin for the High-Fat dinners but still experienced high blood glucose levels. The study lasted for forty-eight hours. It was a closed-loop study. That is, no exercise was allowed, and they ate identical amounts of carbohydrates and protein. The only difference between the meals was the amount of fat in them. Another difference was the amount of insulin they took—more for the high-fat meals; by even doing that, they experienced more hyperglycemia. More insulin is needed when people with Type 1 diabetes eat higher-fat meals, according to this research. A researcher wrote, "Our findings are consistent with those of previous studies indicating that higher-fat pizza meals cause late after meal (postprandial) hyperglycemia necessitating increased insulin doses. The time course of the increase in the glucose concentrations after the higher-fat dinner meal is in keeping with studies in nondiabetic humans indicating that physiological Free Fatty Acids elevations lead to insulin resistance within several hours."[58]

Eating saturated fat like in a hamburger also changes the timing of the rise in blood glucose after a meal. Fat takes up to six hours to move through the gastrointestinal tract. Whereas rapid-acting insulin such as Novolog, Humalog, or Apidra and the new faster acting insulins Fiasp or Lyumjev (I highly recommend using Fiasp or Lyumjev because they become active in two minutes instead of 15 to 20 like the others) stay active for just four hours. When you eat a high-fat meal, a significant amount of glucose remains after the four-hour life of the rapid-acting insulin. This results in elevated blood glucose readings. For example, Red Robin's Bacon Cheeseburger has 71 grams of total fat, with 24 being saturated. The burger also has 50 grams of carbohydrates. One effective way to combat this is to get your hamburger lettuce wrapped, leaving off the cheese and carbohydrate bun.

The following are the American Heart Association's guidelines for fat consumption: Limit total fat intake to less than 25–35 percent of your total calories daily and limit saturated fat intake to less than 7 percent. This means a 2000-calorie meal plan could include 140 calories from saturated fat, or 16 grams. It is also best not to eat those 16 grams in one sitting.

Reduce consumption of saturated fats like red meat and dairy products. Think chicken, turkey, and almond milk. Monounsaturated fats like olives, avocados, cashews, almonds, peanuts, and olive and peanut oil lower LDL ("bad") cholesterol and insulin resistance and raise HDL. Polyunsaturated fats are found in salmon, herring, tuna, cod, pumpkin, sunflower seeds and oil, and corn oil. They also lower LDL cholesterol and triglyceride levels. Instead of using canola oil which is highly processed, use coconut oil, olive oil, and organic butter. Dr. Axe says, "Despite unjustified warnings about saturated fat from well-meaning, albeit misinformed, experts, the list of butter's benefits is impressive: Butter is full of vitamins, minerals, and MCFA that greatly benefit overall health." However, the amount used in one sitting matters for blood sugar control with carbohydrate consumption.

Avoid meals containing 40 or more grams of fat, especially if the fat is saturated. Alter the amount and timing of your insulin if you eat a high-fat meal, taking an additional smaller dose later, especially if you've eaten some carbohydrates with the meal. For people with Type 2 diabetes, taking oral medications and those on insulin, doing some physical activity—for example, walking after a high-fat meal—can help control blood glucose. And by all means, lower the amount of carbohydrates you eat—15 grams or at most 30 grams per meal. And ideally, with a high-fat meal, avoid carbs altogether.

In summary, these are the steps to take for the key to victory. Avoid meals containing 40 or more grams of fat, especially if the fat is saturated. Please keep it to 16 grams a day or 5 per meal. If you decide to eat pizza, eat the thin-crust kind. One piece has 202 calories, 18 grams of carbohydrates, and 4.3 grams of fat. If you eat a hamburger, eat a lettuce-wrapped one and avoid the carbohydrates altogether. And get some exercise after you eat. Research indicates if people sit after a meal, their blood sugar peaks like a mountain for about two hours. The mountains become safe, gentle rolling hills if people take a 15-minute walk at one mph after a meal. With a one mph walk after a meal, you restrict the blood sugar peaks to half the size. So, if your blood glucose is 100, it will increase by 50 points.

When you eat, eat the vegetables first, then the protein, and finally the carbohydrates. Jessie Inchauspe writes, "The slower the trickling of glucose into our bloodstream, the flatter our glucose curves and the better we feel. We can eat exactly the same thing—but by eating carbs last, we make a big difference in our physical and mental well-being. What's more, when we eat foods in the right order, our pancreas produces less insulin. And as I explained in Part 2, less insulin helps us return to fat-burning mode more quickly, the positive results of which are many—and include losing weight."

For a good explanation of fat watch: What is fat?—George Zaidan" at **https://www.youtube.com/watch?v=QhUrc4BnPgg&t=7s**

14 Fast—Use time-restricted eating in the evening and morning.

"Man eats too much. Thus he lives on only a quarter of what he consumes. The doctors, however, live on the remaining three quarters." (Ancient Egyptian Doctor)

"There are multitudes of diseases which have their origin in fullness, and might have their end in fasting."—James Morrison.

The study in #13, about 420 participants—early and late eaters—also relates to this wise way. The largest meal, with 40 percent of daily calories, was eaten before 3 p.m. or after. The early eaters benefitted most from weight loss and blood glucose control.

Another study called "Early Time-Restricted Eating" at the University of Alabama correlates with early and late eaters' research.[59] They studied overweight people on two different eating schedules. One was eating from 8 am to 8 pm and the other only from 8 am to 2 pm. They discovered that more fat was burned by eating during a smaller window of time, the second category. Their research indicates more fat was burned during the night with fewer food cravings during the day. I've used this idea to eat my last meal earlier in the day and especially to not eat after the last meal! I maintain better blood glucose control when I can follow this schedule. (I'm not always able to do so because my blood sugar levels get too low before bedtime. I can't go to bed with an 80 mg/dl, especially when I know the level will drop.) Do your own research. Try avoiding snacks during the evening and before bed. See if your blood glucose improves.

After trying Time-Restricted Eating in the evenings, you could restrict your eating all morning. In other words, do some fasting until noon or one. Then you would have a window to eat for the next six hours. I've done this successfully for better blood sugar control and weight loss. There are several things to consider when trying an 18:6 or 16:8 (fasting for 16 to 18 hours and having an eating window from six to eight hours) fasting schedule. Sixteen hours may seem long, but if you're getting adequate sleep, you should be asleep for about seven hours. These characteristics, like knowledge, self-control, perseverance, and hope, will apply to fasting.

Let's consider the first one on knowledge. *"Wise people have success by means of great power. Those who have knowledge gather strength"* (Proverbs 24:5 NIRV). Continuing to fast after an evening of Time-Restricted Eating is an easy way to start to fast because you already have a night's head start. During the morning, have no calories that could stimulate insulin and eat food for energy production. When we eat, our energy source comes from carbohydrates, which the body converts into glucose. Any glucose we don't utilize for energy the body converts into glycogen stored in the liver. And if we overeat and our glycogen stores are full, the carbs are converted to fat. How many times a week should you fast for sixteen to eighteen hours? Since I have Type 1 Diabetes, it depends on how I do in the evening. If I've calculated the grams of carbohydrates and the insulin I take and my blood glucose keeps from getting low, I can fast. I watch my blood glucose with my continuous glucose monitor and lower my basal dose.

However, if you have type 1 diabetes, it is important to remember that ketone levels may rise when you are not eating. This may be a challenge if you need more basal insulin and depend on meal-time insulin to avoid high levels of ketones. The good news is that you can measure your ketone levels. It is also essential to monitor blood glucose levels—hypoglycemia is a risk of fasting.

Benjamin Horne, M.D. gives this caution for those with Type 2 Diabetes on medications. "If you are taking medications that are aimed at reducing the amount of glucose in your blood, together with fasting these can cause potentially fatal hypoglycemia," Horne says. "It's not a minor safety risk." So, consult your healthcare team before trying this if you are on medications to control your blood glucose levels.

The second point is it takes self-control during the morning hours to fast. *"Like a city whose walls are broken through is a person who lacks self-control"* (Proverbs 25:28). City walls were defense mechanisms for ancient cities to defend themselves and keep enemies out. Since many people have breakfast during the morning, how can they manage the hunger pains? By drinking water and other no-calorie beverages, like plain coffee or tea. You will be surprised at how you can ward off hunger pangs.

Another thing we need to do during those morning hours is not succumb to temptations. Keep snack food out of reach and out of sight. By doing this, you can persevere and reap great rewards for your health. *"Let us not become weary in doing good, for at the proper time we will reap a harvest if we do not give up"* (Galatians 6:9). What is happening with your body as you fast? It helps to know so that you can endure and not give up. Here is a basic outline of what I've read happens. For the first eight hours, blood sugars fall, food has left the stomach, and the body produces minimal insulin for basal metabolisms like breathing and the heart. Does your BMR stop working during sickness? "The basal metabolic rate, or BMR is the amount of energy required to support the work of the heart, brain, lungs, and other organs at rest, in the absence of any physical or mental exertion," says Boris Draznin, M.D. Then, for the next four hours, the digestive system sleeps, the body begins healing, and human growth hormone increases. During hours twelve through eighteen, this is what happens.

Food consumed has been burned, the digestive system goes to sleep, the body begins the healing process, human growth hormone begins to increase, and glucagon is relaxed to balance blood sugars during the twelve and thirteenth hours. After fourteen hours, the body has converted to using stored fat as energy, and human growth hormone starts to increase dramatically.[60] **This means that after fourteen hours of fasting, you start losing fat weight, not muscle.**

Here are six benefits of having increased growth hormone: Increased muscle strength, better fracture healing, enhanced weight loss, stronger bones, reduced heart disease risk, and better mood and sleep. After fourteen hours of fasting, the body begins to use stored fat as energy, and after sixteen hours, it begins to ramp up the fat burning.

To lose weight, have you ever experienced your body having a plateau effect? You get to a certain weight loss, and then you can't seem to lose another pound? This is where fasting is so beneficial. Instead of your fat-burning rate slowing down to conserve energy, it ramps up. One research study showed an increase of 12%.

Following an intermittent fasting diet can make maintaining the weight you lost over the long term easier. A two-part study of 40 obese adults, published in Frontiers in Physiology in 2016, compared the combined effects of a high-protein, low-kilojoule (foods such as fruits, vegetables, and legumes are less energy-dense foods), intermittent-fasting diet plan with a traditional heart-healthy diet plan. The results showed that while both diets proved to be equally successful in reductions in body mass index (BMI) and blood lipids (fatty acids and cholesterol), those on the intermittent-fasting diet showed an advantage in minimizing weight regain after one year.

So here is another benefit called hope, not wishful thinking. *"Hope deferred makes the heart sick, but a longing fulfilled is a tree of life"* Proverbs 13:12. One person in our diabetes meetings uses intermittent fasting daily and needs a new wardrobe because of weight loss. I call that hope, not just wishful thinking. **Fasting works for a healthier life!**

What Is a Secret Weight Loss Weapon?

If we have the proper levels of this hormone, it will help us enjoy a healthier lifestyle, especially if we have Type 2 Diabetes and want to lose weight. It is a secret weight loss weapon. We don't have direct control over it like you do with your leg and arm muscles, but we can affect its production indirectly. What is this secret weapon? It is a secret because have you heard of adiponectin? Two hormones produced in white fat cells can enhance weight loss: adiponectin and leptin (feel full hormone). Adiponectin will boost your body's metabolism, help your cells' sensitivity to insulin, and increase your muscles' conversion of glucose for energy. It will also enhance the quicker breakdown of fat for energy, which is called fat oxidation. Adiponectin helps with this process during fasting.[61]

Adiponectin acts on various receptors, increasing skeletal muscle and liver fatty acid oxidation. Adiponectin levels decrease in proportion to the accumulation of visceral fat. A beneficial effect of intermittent fasting is the shift during fasting from glucose or glycogen to fatty acids as the fuel source. When we practice intermittent fasting, we reduce adiposity, that is, the condition of having excessive body fat or obesity. Because of this reduction in too much fat, patients may experience improvements in their leptin/adiponectin levels and sensitivity, resulting in improved appetite control.

This process primarily occurs in the cell's mitochondria

and is vital to the body's energy metabolism. Saturated fat is a known cause of insulin resistance. The more sensitive our body is to insulin, the better our blood glucose control will be. Efficient amounts of adiponectin play a significant role in our body's insulin sensitivity. One type of fat that many people carry is visceral fat, which is a significant contributor to insulin resistance and lower levels of adiponectin.

"Be sure you know the condition of your flocks, give careful attention to your herds" (Proverbs 27:23). So what does this have to do with our health? The principle of this wisdom teaching is to know the condition of what you own, which would include your health. In other words, keeping track of what you eat is a good idea.

Tails up or tails down is one way to differentiate between sheep and goats. A goat usually holds its tail up unless it is sick or injured. Sheep tails hang down. I don't have any flocks. But again, it is also appropriate to consider what you do, including what you eat and how much exercise you get. *"The wisdom of the prudent is to give thought to their ways"* (Proverbs 14: 8). *"The simple believe anything, but the prudent give thought to their steps"* (Proverbs 14: 15). Wisdom also teaches about how much you eat, self-control, and portion control when eating.

It's not enough to simply say, "I enjoy eating some popcorn or chips each evening." We must ask ourselves, how much is too much? Similarly, saying, "I try to get a little exercise each day," is a good start, but we should be curious about how much exercise is truly beneficial. And when it comes to carbs, it's not enough to say we're cutting back. We should be willing to learn about the impact of carbs on our health.

Can we boost our adiponectin levels through our diet and exercise? Absolutely. Both methods can be beneficial. A review and analysis of 22 trials involving 2,996 individuals showed that physical exercise, particularly aerobic exercise, increased adiponectin levels in prediabetic and diabetic adults.

According to one study, legume consumption increases adiponectin among type 2 diabetic patients. This clinical trial investigated the effects of substituting legumes for meat consumption in a lifestyle change diet on leptin and adiponectin amounts among type 2 diabetic patients. Researchers randomly assigned thirty-one type 2 diabetic patients (24 women, age: 58.1±6.0 years) to groups designated to consume a legume-free diet or a bean (legume-based) diet for eight weeks. Both diets were similar except for replacing two servings of red meat with legumes, that is, beans, three days per week in the legume-based group. Leptin and adiponectin concentrations were measured at baseline and after eight weeks. The legume-based diet significantly increased adiponectin amounts in comparison with the legume-free diet. There was no significant change in leptin amounts after both intervention diets.

In conclusion, Legumes or beans increase adiponectin in type 2 diabetic patients. What other values do beans provide? Beans are an excellent, affordable source of protein, fiber, and minerals. Adding beans to a meal can help people keep their blood sugar levels stable and help keep the body healthy.

To encourage your body to produce more adiponectin, incorporate more foods rich in omega-3 fatty acids, such as salmon, sardines, tuna, chia seeds, and flaxseed, and other delicious monounsaturated fats like avocados, nuts, olives, and olive oil into your diet. Berries, such as blueberries and straw-berries, legumes or beans, and vegetables, such as spinach, kale, and broccoli, are also known to boost its production.[62] Inflammation in joints, arteries, and muscles can make life painful. When you have chronic inflammation, the extra pressure your body is under makes daily tasks, such as standing, walking, and bending, more painful. The rich antioxidants found in blueberries, along with some vital nutrients such as Manganese, can help your body repair and reduce inflammation. Blueberries also feed the usefulness of adiponectin.

Again, adiponectin will boost your body's metabolism, help your cells' sensitivity to insulin, and increase your muscles' conversion of glucose for energy. It will also enhance the quicker breakdown of fat for energy, which is called fat oxidation. Adiponectin helps with this process during fasting. **Greater levels of adiponectin result in improved appetite control. So, exercise more and increase your intake of beans and other whole foods to increase your levels of adiponectin.**

15 Have a good night's sleep.

"My son, do not let wisdom and understanding out of your sight...When you lie down, you will not be afraid; when you lie down, your sleep will be sweet... When you walk, they will guide you; when you sleep, they will watch over you; when you awake, they will speak to you. (Proverbs 3:21, 24; 6:22).

Some people claim they can get by with just four or five hours of sleep per night. How many hours of sleep are needed? The Centers for Disease Control recommends, along with the Mayo Clinic, no less than seven hours a night. Many people aren't getting enough sleep. One in three adults reports they sleep an average of six or fewer hours a night.[63] The average sleep of the millions of people using Fitbit health-trackers is only six-hours and thirty-eight minutes per night.[64] Drowsy driving is an ever-present dangerous result of sleep deprivation. According to the Centers for Disease Control, an estimated one in twenty-five adult drivers reports falling asleep while driving in the previous 30 days. Drowsy driving is also estimated to cause 72,000 crashes, 44,000 injuries, and 800 deaths in 2013. These numbers are underestimated, and up to 6,000 fatal crashes each year may be caused by drowsy drivers.[65]

Physical health is also impacted by sleep deprivation. There is an impairment of hormones that relate to appetite. Less leptin, the "feel full" hormone is released, and more of ghrelin, the "still hungry" hormone. This makes losing weight an even greater challenge. So, the strategy is to sleep more and lose weight.[66] Studies also reveal that cortisol levels increase the next evening after just one night of sleep loss, causing insulin resistance. Also, the efficiency of the immune response is damaged as well as an increase in inflammation with lack of sleep.[67] A lack of sleep also lowers the levels of the chemical serotonin, which then results in pain sensitivity increasing as well as increased feelings of anxiety. To compensate for lower levels, the body compensates with cravings for carbohydrates.[68]

When we sleep, we are not just dreaming and wasting time. Our bodies are designed to use that time to stay or get healthy! Several processes are happening as we sleep. According to the National Sleep Foundation, such health benefits as "muscle repair, memory consolidation and release of hormones regulating growth and appetite" are happening. This prepares us to concentrate and make decisions for all day time activities. As we sleep, we go through several stages of sleep. These stages repeat throughout the night in about ninety-minute cycles. Our bodies are as the psalmist writes, *"Fearfully and wonderfully made"* (Psalm 139:14).

Fitbit health trackers have divided sleep into three stages—light, deep and REM sleep. Imagine a maintenance crew working during the light stage. During light sleep, body maintenance is at work keeping a perfect balance, a homeostasis of all bodily functions and hormones. Light sleep is important because it comprises about 50% of sleep each night. With the lack of sleep, several hormones that affect weight will not be in balance such as leptin, ghrelin, cortisol, and growth hormone.[69]

During normal sleep, the metabolic rate is reduced by about 15%. The amount of energy (calories) the body burns to maintain itself is metabolism. That is why my basal rate of insulin in my insulin pump is so low compared to other times of the day—.30 units per hour compared to .90 at breakfast time. I don't need as much energy to supply my needs thus less insulin is needed during the night.[70]

Picture a person's tense arm muscles holding up a shield to deflect incoming harmful arrows. During deep sleep, the immune system is strengthened. Growth hormone is secreted which results in cellular rebuilding and repair. This is also the time the body uses for muscle development.

Also, picture a profile of a person's brain with colorful lights going off within the brain. Processing and storing information happens during the REM (rapid eye movement) stage of sleep. Vivid dreams occur, the body is relaxed and the volunteer skeletal muscles are turned off. Maybe that prevents acting out those vivid dreams. If deep sleep is about the body, REM sleep is about the brain. Mental restoration is taking place so that you can clearly think and decide during the day.[71]

How do you wake up after a night's sleep? Are you groggy and feel like you haven't slept or do you wake up refreshed? I've found my Fitbit Health tracker very beneficial for keeping me aware of the kind of sleep I'm getting. It also identifies how much of the night I'm awake too. This helps me plan my schedule for when to go to bed and when to get up so I can get an adequate amount of sleep. *"The plans of the diligent lead to profit (health) as surely as haste leads to poverty"* (Proverbs 21:5).

Certain foods help promote sleep. The Institute of Health Sciences recommends foods that contain tryptophan, which helps induce the production of serotonin, which is required to make melatonin.[72] Melatonin is a hormone that regulates sleep-wake cycles. The body produces more during darkness, preparing the body for sleep. Light has the reverse effect.[73]

Foods that help with this are grass-fed dairy products, nuts, fish, chicken, turkey, sprouted grains, beans and brown rice, eggs, sesame seeds, and sunflower seeds. Eat melatonin-rich foods like bananas, Morello cherries, ginger, barley, tomatoes, and radishes. Include them in your dinner or supper. For a complete discussion on getting to sleep, go to Dr. Josh Axe's (a certified doctor of natural medicine) article "Top 20 Ways to Fall Asleep Fast!"[74]

Difficulty Falling to Sleep?

Why? Jesus himself took naps. Remember what happened on the Sea of Galilee? *"A furious squall came up, and the waves broke over the boat, so that it was nearly swamped. Jesus was in the stern, sleeping on a cushion"* (Mark 4:37-38). What is amazing about this event is that Jesus was sleeping during a storm. Have you ever had difficulty falling asleep? All of us have, but Jesus could sleep even during a storm. How?

God's wisdom gives us a key. *"Do not let wisdom and under-standing out of your sight...Then you will go on your way in safety, and your foot will not stumble. When you lie down, you will not be afraid; when you lie down, your sleep will be sweet"* (Proverbs 3:22-24). *"When you walk, they will guide you; when you sleep, they will watch over you; when you awake, they will speak to you"* (Proverbs 6:22).

Have you ever had a root canal done? The procedure can be excruciating. How do you handle the pain? Meditation helps. I've gone over and over in my mind calming words like *"God is my shield and refuge"* from Proverbs 30:5. *"Every word of God is flawless; he is a shield to those who take refuge in him."* Positive wise thinking can bring a calming effect to a stressful situa-tion. *"Be careful what you think, because your thoughts run your life"* (Proverbs 4:23 NCV). By doing this we keep in our sight wisdom and understanding, which we read brings sweet sleep. *"Whoever seeks good finds favor, but evil comes to one who searches for it"* (Proverbs 11:27). By seeking what is good, listing the good, meditating on the good are all practices of keeping wisdom in sight. These are all methods for having sweet sleep. And we are talking about Jesus' wisdom.

What can easily happen instead of focusing on the good is to focus on problems or worries. Thinking about them over and over again is not conducive to falling asleep. In fact, by meditating on them they are compounded and become independent of reality. These worries can easily become worse and more powerful than they are. This all leads to restlessness and mounting obstacles and hazards for falling asleep. Dwelling on what is good will fight off the anxiety of worry. *"A cheerful look brings joy to your heart. And good news gives health to your body"* (Proverbs 15:30 NIrV).

A ten-week research study with hundreds of participants was done by Professor Robert Emmons, Ph.D., while he taught at the University of California at Davis to demonstrate what effects gratitude might have on health and well-being. They were randomly divided into three groups. One group was a gratitude condition group, and the members were to list five things for which they could be thankful that had affected their lives from the previous week. Another group was the hassle group, and those people were to list five burdens that affected their lives the previous week. The third group was the neutral group, and its members were to list five things, either positive or negative, that had affected their lives the previous week.

The results were then analyzed with several tests. The final analysis was that the people in the gratitude group felt better about their lives, were more optimistic, and exercised more than those in the other groups. The results were even better when gratitude was practiced daily, looking at a variety of blessings.[75]

Several other studies have been conducted with similar results. For example, another ten-week study was done by the Department of Physical Medicine and Rehabilitation at the University of Cal-Davis, involving people with post-polio syndrome. The results of the gratitude group were that the people felt better about themselves, felt more optimistic about the coming week, and felt more connected with others than the other groups. Another significant finding was that they went to sleep quicker, spent more time sleeping, and felt more refreshed in the morning.[76] **The idea is that if you want to sleep more soundly, count your blessings, not sheep.**

16 Correct low-blood glucose: hypoglycemia. Outsmart Hypoglycemia—Eat Smarties®

According to Proverbs 24:14, people have hope when they find wisdom, which inspires them not to give up. *"Wisdom is sweet to your soul. If you find it, there is a future hope for you, and your hope will not be cut off."* God's wisdom applies in the following way—to give thought to managing diabetes. *"The wisdom of the prudent is to give thought to their ways...The prudent see danger and take refuge"* (Proverbs 14:8, 22:3).

One of the dangers of diabetes is hypoglycemia. In the "Diabetes Attitudes, Wishes and Needs" research study, researchers found a deep fear of hypoglycemia (blood glucose levels below 70 mg/dl).[77] These episodes can happen at any time during the day. So, being prudent and alert is essential. Hypoglycemia is an acute stress factor for people using insulin or Sulfonylurea medications like Glipizide or Glyburide. Blood glucose can get low when too much insulin is in circulation. Epinephrine (adrenaline) is the "fight or flight" hormone that alerts the body to danger or stressful situations. It produces symptoms of low blood glucose like weakness, hunger, sweating, trembling, "butterflies," and heart palpitations. Epinephrine activates Glucagon. Glucagon releases stored glucose or glycogen in the liver, raising blood glucose levels (glycogenolysis). A person without diabetes might experience some of these symptoms if they haven't eaten for several hours. What I just described are the usual responses for people without diabetes. Still, the normal responses are compromised for those with Type 1 Diabetes or Type 2 on insulin or medications like Glipizide because too much insulin may be in circulation. So, taking carbohydrates to raise the blood sugar level is essential to prevent dangerous lows.

The epinephrine response gets blunted for many people who have had Type 1 diabetes for many years. They lose the early warning signs of low blood glucose. Lower and lower blood glucose levels have to occur before their response occurs. So, instead of being in the 60's mg/dl blood glucose levels, it may be less than 40 mg/dl. According to the Joslin Diabetes Center, new research indicates that avoiding hypoglycemia episodes can restore the proper, timely response of the epinephrine, giving the warning signs at a much higher, safer blood glucose level.[78]

A great precaution is to check our blood glucose more often. When not using my continuous glucose monitoring system,

I check myself up to twelve times daily. Regularly checking yourself is essential, especially if you are on insulin or the medications previously mentioned. This reduces the risk of having a severe episode! Another precaution is always having glucose tablets, Smarties®, or SweeTarts® with you. For a visual episode of not taking this precaution while on a walk, watch "Jim's 1st Person Low" at **https://www.youtube.com/ watch?v=f7SEaZSWqXs**

How many grams of quick-energy carbohydrates are needed to treat low blood glucose readings? A good rule of thumb is that 1 gram of glucose raises the blood sugar by 3, 4, or 5 points for body weights of 200, 150, or 100 pounds, respectively. For example, 5 grams of dextrose, as found in Smarties® or SweeTarts®, raises the blood sugar by about 20 points for a 150-lb person.[79]

Treat a low with 15 grams of Smarties® or similar candy, then wait twenty minutes and check again. Also, combine a low glycemic index carbohydrate with a fast-acting carbohydrate. For example, I woke up one night at about 2 am to visit the restroom. I checked my blood glucose and discovered it was 46 mg/ dl. So, I took 9 grams of Smarties® (GI of 96) and a small amount of milk (6 grams of carb—GI of 34). When I checked my blood glucose at 6 am, I was 116. Since I weigh about 150 lbs. the 15 grams of carbs should have elevated my blood glucose by 60 points. That number and the combination of carbs increased my blood glucose level by 70 points. Measuring the amount of carbohydrates will prevent overcompensating and ending up with high blood glucose!

As a preventive for hypoglycemia at night, check your blood glucose right before bed. If you take insulin, always know how much insulin is active (Humalog and NovoLog last for four hours). This plan has worked for me in the 64+ years I've had diabetes, preventing ambulance calls and hospitalization (only once in 1991).

17 Take advantage of opportunities to help others. To Be Encouraged, Encourage

"A good person gives life to others; the wise person teaches others how to live" (Proverbs 11:30 NCV).

Glenn lived by himself (He had LADA diabetes for twenty years—Latent Autoimmune Diabetes in Adults, a progressively slow-developing Type 1 with his beta-producing insulin cells being destroyed). He picked up a business card at the local pharmacy for the diabetes support group. He started attending the meetings. He encouraged and received support from others who were also facing many of the same challenges with diabetes.

"A generous person will prosper; whoever refreshes others will be refreshed" (Proverbs 11:25). He put this wisdom into practice. He became very involved with the community diabetes support group. When several of us would meet to count advertising flyers for a diabetes seminar to mail, he would be there! He knew people would attend because they received one of the mailed flyers. And they would be helped to control their diabetes. He would set up chairs in the large community room at the library for seminar participants. He was helping, being encouraged, and encouraging!

Blood glucose control was a perpetual struggle for him. God

has marvellously designed the human body. When we eat carbohydrates, they reach the small intestine, a hormone (GLP1), a messenger, goes to the pancreas and signals for an initial release of stored insulin and manufacturing more. The amount is exact to meet the needs of the number of carbohydrates eaten and will keep the blood glucose in a tight range between 70 to 140 mg/dl. But people like Glenn do not have the beta cells that produce insulin. His body has destroyed them. He required a strict balancing act, which is a great challenge! Someone said that managing diabetes is like playing the piano with your right hand while juggling with your left hand, all while trying to keep your balance as you walk on a tightrope. Managing diabetes is a balancing act!

All Glenn had to do was take his insulin at the right time, in just the right amount, several times each day; check his blood sugars multiple times a day to make sure he wasn't too high or too low; balance the right amount of food with the insulin he took. Stay alert for stress or colds that elevate the stress hormone cortisol causing elevated blood sugars. And also realize he must do this every day because there is never a vacation from diabetes. That's how simple it can be! Ha! People like Glenn need encouragement! We all need to give help and receive help!

There is nothing like experiencing a low, low blood sugar. An extremely low reading is like squeezing out every ounce or milligram of glucose to stay conscious. I've experienced this nightmare situation several times but have stayed conscious. Glenn's blood glucose was a rollercoaster of ups and downs. I called him one afternoon, asking how he was doing. He was out of blood glucose checking strips. He had been having lows, and some were extremely low. I told him my wife, and I would bring him some strips. We found him on his bedroom floor, helpless, sitting with his legs crossed in briefs. His eyes were glazed. He barely recognized me.

Immediately I checked his blood glucose. It was about 20 mg/dl. This was a severe hypoglycemic episode. The race was on to keep him conscious. Since he was awake and could swallow, I gave him Smarties® from my glucose-checking kit. The Smarties® eventually brought him out of the severe low. Ten days later, he suffered another severe episode. No one was there to help, and he died. Many people need a helping hand. Many have helped me—my wife, parents, friends, doctors, and nurses. One morning I woke up with stickiness on the back of my head—honey. I was so distressingly in a severe hypoglycemic episode I would not cooperate. So my wife put honey on my lips, which eventually saved me. Each day let's think about helping others.

God's wisdom applies in the following way: to think about what we do. *"The wisdom of the prudent is to give thought to their ways...The prudent see danger and take refuge"* (Proverbs 14:8, 22:3). A great precaution we all can take is to check our blood glucose more often. The other practice is to keep focused on helping others. Not only will they benefit, but we will too!

> *"Two are better than one, because they have a good return for their labor: If either of them falls down, one can help the other up. But pity anyone who falls and has no one to help them up."* (Ecclesiastes 4:9-10)

Remember when you were in school? Were you comfortable

sitting with your friends at lunchtime? Or, do you remember lunchtime being a time you dreaded because you sat alone? Sitting by yourself is lonely and uncomfortable, especially when everyone else seems to be laughing and enjoying the company of friends. How many new kids sitting alone may think they are the objects of laughter?

Long ago, I heard a professor share this interesting saying: "It's not what I think that's important; it's not what you think that is important, but it's what I think you think that's important." There are usually no lunchtime welcoming committees for new kids! Most students or teenagers show little concern about new people. *"A person who isn't friendly looks out only for himself"* (Proverbs 18:1). How true that proverb is at lunchtime in many schools.

At Boca High School in Florida, the "We Dine Together" group abruptly halted an ordinary lunchtime. Denis Estimon and three other students began the year determined not to let anyone eat alone unless they wanted to. This started during Denis's senior year, but he remembered being lonely as an immigrant first-grader. Dozens are now members of a high school of 3,400 students. Other schools have initiated "We Dine Together" clubs.[80] Those in their 50s who remember how it was growing up are expressing their comments of appreciation for what they are doing. They told their appreciation with such comments as "lunch periods were achingly uncomfortable" or "I walked instead of ate lunch." One mother discovered her son suffered so much social isolation that he would hide while eating.

What would Jesus do? He taught, *"Do to others as you would have them do to you"* (Luke 6:31). Jesus reached out to socially isolated people—lepers, tax collectors, and the sick. He even ate with tax collectors, who were avoided and ridiculed by others. Jesus knew kindness and attention were greatly appreciated. Paul wrote, *"Always try to be kind to each other and to everyone else...clothe yourselves with compassion, kindness, humility, gentleness and patience...whoever refreshes others will be refreshed...goodwill is found among the upright"* (1 Thessalonians 5:15, Colossians 3:12, Proverbs 11:25, 14:9).

These teenagers are practicing God's wisdom in a wonderfully kind way! "We Dine Together" clubs run in every state and even Canada.

Watch: "So no student eats alone" at **https://www.youtube.com/watch?v=lfIl5Rw6dBQ** and **https://www.facebook.com/wedinetogether/**

Let's not let others suffer alone. Let's support others because God is helping us with his wisdom. I started a Diabetes Education and Support group in the fall of 1992 and continue to start one wherever I live. God gives us tremendous power through his wisdom to overcome, be resilient, and persevere even with Diabetes and illness! So, let's help others; as we do so, we help ourselves! *"The wise prevail through great power, and those who have knowledge muster their strength...For the LORD gives wisdom; from his mouth come knowledge and understanding. He holds success in store for the upright... Do not let them out of your sight, keep them within your heart; for they are life to those who find them and health to one's whole body"* (Proverbs 24:5, 2:7-8, 4:21-22).

Part 2
Common Sense Guidelines for Living Well with Diabetes

CHAPTER FOUR

Be Motivated

Over one million people have viewed it in just seven days, with more than 1,300 comments. That was three years ago, but now there have been more than 7.2 million views and over 3,500 comments, which shows its popularity. What is it? A video of "Momma Bear Struggles with Cubs." We can learn essential Biblical principles from this scene, like this passage.

"All the days of the oppressed are wretched, but the cheerful heart has a continual feast" (Proverbs 15:15). How are a continual feast and a cheerful heart connected? One way to have a merry heart is to focus on things that bring cheer. So a story that gave joy to my heart concerned a mother bear with her four cubs.

She stops traffic on a highway with her escapades. Her goal is to cross this highway with her uncooperative cubs. Her first step to get across is picking up one of the cubs by the nape of his neck while another trots joyfully behind her. The other two don't bother to follow. After a few seconds, one of them, not seeing his mother, begins in a cute trot to cross the highway alone. (This entire story was playing out as traffic was backing up.) The last cub refuses to cross the road and instead starts climbing the tree. That climb doesn't last long because Mom comes running across the highway to get him, and again one of the other cubs has to follow her. She grabs him off the tree by the nape of the neck while the other cub scrambles under her feet. They start but get halfway when she drops that cub and goes after the other one. The trouble is that the first one does not stay where he is dropped but begins to follow her. (We are now seventy-three seconds into this effort.) She struggles with the cubs for about twenty seconds. Finally, she picks up one of them and begins to run. The other cub gets the clue to follow. She drops that first one, but it begins to go back to the original side. Finally, here comes Mom, who grabs the cub again and scurries safely across the highway.

Several words describe this situation: frustration, uncooperative, determination, persistence, patience, devotion, and humor. This mother/cub interaction happens in only 123 seconds, to be exact. Watch "Momma Bear Struggles with Cubs" at https://www.youtube.com/watch?v=ho3IFJiBzrY&t=63s

Why did I share this story? Like that mother bear, it reminds me of how frustrating it can be to do all the things necessary to keep my blood glucose or sugar near the normal range.

"I'm discouraged, feel lousy, and just can't seem to do what I need to do." Do you ever experience feelings like that? Yet, motivation is needed to walk more, count carbohydrates, check blood sugar, and avoid foods that drive up blood sugar. What motivates you?

Does avoiding long-term diabetes complications like blindness, amputation, foot pain from peripheral neuropathy, kidney failure, and heart disease motivate you to conquer diabetes? Does that fear motivate you to "go get it done" to control your blood sugars today? Or are you like I thought? Complications are what other people experience, not me. Besides, the possibilities of complications are in the distant future, not today.

When looking at the challenges of controlling diabetes, why not focus on feeling better today? If I feel better today, I can avoid or lower the risk of complications, help others do the same, look and be healthy, continue to enjoy the company of those I love—friends, family, and grandchildren, and do the right things by developing healthy habits!

The following quote is uplifting because it speaks of the expectation of success. *"For the LORD gives wisdom; from his mouth come knowledge and understanding. He holds success (or victory) in store for the upright"* (Proverbs 2:7-8). So, when I do everything needed to outsmart diabetes with this resource, success will be the result. That is motivational; it helps us focus on the goal of victory. And God gives his wisdom for us to succeed, to have victory for health and wellness. God cares about us! *"My son, pay attention to what I say; turn your ear to my words. Do not let them out of your sight, keep them within your heart; for they are life to those who find them and **health to one's whole body**"* (Proverbs 4:20-22).

I included seventeen wise ways to outsmart diabetes from the resource of God's wisdom. They are common-sense approaches for everything needed to manage this disease that is underrated, insidious, but deadly. The following example shows the importance of motivation after a horrendous accident. It is the kind of motivation we can all practice.

After Tragedy

Facing tragedy is difficult, especially because it could change everything about a person's life. This happened to a Mayo Clinic ER Doctor. As he was biking with a friend and riding over a hill, the next thing he knew, he was looking up at a group of concerned people. He had a strange numb feeling around his waist. When he tried to move his legs, they wouldn't respond. He spent the next four and a half months learning wheelchair basics, like how to get in and out of his wheelchair without falling.

After this disaster, he knew of only two choices about what he would do with his life. He knew he was going to do something about his paralysis, or he was going to sit and wallow in self-pity. He chose the first and was back at work five months after the accident.

This doctor believes being in a wheelchair has made him a better physician. He would tower over people with his six-foot, five-inch height, but now he is on their level. He thinks his conversations have become much more understanding with patients. For example, he has a typical patient-doctor interaction when he asks questions and orders blood work. Then he pulls back the curtain and reveals that both the patient and doctor are in wheelchairs.

What drives him on? Being a physician is what he's always wanted to be. He smiles and considers it his privilege to practice medicine and to help influence the lives of others. He knows he could have died.[81]

We see in the story of Doctor David Grossman how important having the attitude to overcome obstacles is. God's wisdom states, *"If you are wise, your wisdom will reward you"* (Proverbs

9:12). How was God's wisdom rewarding him? He didn't give up. He had the attitude to overcome. *"The spirit of a man will sustain him in sickness, but who can bear a broken spirit?"* (Proverbs 18:14 NKJV). We also see how valuable compassionately relating to others is. Peter wrote in his first letter, *"Finally, all of you, be like-minded, **be sympathetic,** love one another, be **compassionate** and humble"* (1 Peter 3:8).

As I read this story, I thought about how understanding Jesus, our great physician, is with us. Jesus not only knew about the struggles and hardships people face, but **he experienced them himself.** The author of Hebrews wrote, *"Although Jesus was the Son [of God], he learned to be obedient **through his sufferings"*** (Hebrews 5:8). The good news is God gives us his wisdom to overcome tragedy and have victory in life (Read Proverbs 2:6-7).

Watch: "ER Physician Forms Stronger Bond with Patients after Tragedy | NBC Nightly News" at **https://www.youtube. com/watch?v=gaV4tsrc_JA**

Internal Health Dialogue Prescription for People with Diabetes
When I look at people who struggle with their diabetes to control their blood sugars, I know from my own experience that "it's not as easy as it looks." So, I want to make it easier with tips and ideas from my personal experience as well as research. We need the motivation to do the right things which we can build with God's wisdom! As you continue to read this book, you will notice how God's wisdom intricately applies to life's situations and how that wisdom directly relates to our health. What I experience each day illustrates how Proverbs and wisdom are relevant.

When I get up in the morning, the first thing on my mind is blood sugar. What is my blood glucose level? Is it high, low, or is it just right? So, I check my blood glucose first thing in the morning. Then throughout the day, those thoughts stay with me. After eating lunch, I wonder if I took enough insulin for the carbohydrates I ate. If I'm not wearing my continuous glucose monitor sensor, I'm checking what my blood sugar is. So, I check myself multiple times a day, think about the amount of exercise I'm getting and the number of grams of carbohydrates I'm eating.

I do this to make sure I'm getting the proper balance of food, activity, and insulin to maintain blood sugar levels as close to normal as possible. Do I succeed? Not always. You may think—what an annoyance, nuisance, or hassle! Is that any way to live a life? Yes, because planning a day this way is the "way of wisdom." Proverbs 4:23 states, *"Be careful what you think, because your thoughts run your life."* These are pleasant words or thoughts, and God's wisdom states, *"Pleasant words are like honey. They are sweet to the spirit and bring healing to the body"* (Proverbs 16:24).

Living this way doesn't mean I'm thinking of nothing else. If you are not thinking about your health, though, what you are eating, how many steps you're taking, then start. It is the "way of wisdom." And as I've mentioned, wisdom is "the skill for living."

> *"Keep their words in mind forever as though you had them tied around your neck. They will guide you when you walk. They will guard you when you sleep. They will speak to you when you are awake"* (Proverbs 6:21-22).

CHAPTER FIVE

Use God's Wisdom, The Power of Optimism

WW2 Example

The following story illustrates optimism's power—how can we endure overwhelming difficulties and survive with victory? It also shows the importance of **Wise Way number 17— taking advantage of opportunities to help others.**

At the end of World War II, the condition of prisoners in concentration camps was horrific. American soldiers were assigned to give medical help to the newly liberated prisoners. George Ritchie was one of the soldiers assigned to a team to do this. He described it as the most shattering experience he had yet had, seeing "the effects of slow starvation, to walk through those barracks where thousands of men had died a little bit at a time over a period of years." The paperwork alone was staggering in trying to relocate these people whose families and even hometowns had disappeared. His team came across one of the prisoners who could help. He obviously hadn't been there long: his posture was erect, his eyes bright, his energy unending. Since he was fluent in English, French, German, Russian, and Polish, he became a kind of unofficial camp translator. His compassion for his fellow prisoners glowed on his face, and it was to this glow that Ritchie would turn when his own spirits were low.

Ritchie was astonished when this man's papers came before him for processing. He had been there since 1939! Ritchie says, "For six years he had lived on the same starvation diet, slept in the same airless and disease-ridden barracks as everyone else, but without the least physical or mental deterioration." "It's not easy for some of them to forgive," Ritchie commented one day as they sat over mugs of tea in the processing center. He said, "So many of them have lost members of their families." Hatred among them ran high toward the Germans. Then, for the first time, he spoke of himself, his wife, two daughters, and three little boys. He told how he and his family lived in the Jewish section of Warsaw and how when the Germans came, they lined up everyone, including his family. He begged to die with his family, but because he spoke German, they put him in a workgroup.

He said, "I had to decide right then whether to let myself hate the soldiers who had done this." His decision was easy, though, because, in his practice as a lawyer, he had already seen what hate could do to people's lives. Hate had just killed his family. He said, "I decided then that I would spend the rest of my life—whether it was a few days or many years—loving every person I came in contact with."[82]

What kept this man thriving while being confronted with every privation? Love is what kept him well! Love is an attribute of God's wisdom. The following are two proverbs of God's wisdom concerning love: *"Hatred stirs up conflict, but love covers over all wrongs"* (Proverbs 10:12). *"Whoever would foster love covers over an offense, but whoever repeats the matter separates close friends"* (Proverbs 17:9). By practicing these two proverbs, they empowered him to endure. If he could live through such horrible circumstances, surely we can meet the challenges we may face daily with diabetes! And we can do so with God's wisdom! *"Choose my instruction instead of silver, knowledge rather than choice gold, for wisdom is more precious than rubies, and nothing you desire can compare with her"* (Proverbs 8:10-11).

More Valuable than Rubies

A man was stunned and overjoyed when an appraiser valued his blanket at an Antique Roadshow. The blanket is considered one of the Roadshow's "Greatest Finds!" The episode starts with an appraiser, Donald Ellis asking the owner to tell him what he knows about the blanket. He didn't know much except that Kit Carson was supposed to have given it to the foster father of his grandmother. He thought it was a Navajo blanket and had never had it appraised. "Ted, did you notice that when you showed this to me, I stopped breathing a little bit," said the appraiser. "It's a chief's blanket, a Ute First Phase wearing blanket. The Navajo's made it from about 1840 to 1860. They were very valuable at that time. This is Navajo weaving in its purest form." Then he was told its condition was "unbelievable."

He had seen nothing so important on the Roadshow. Ted did not have a clue about its value. He was then asked, "Are you a wealthy man?" No! A shocked, overwhelming reaction followed when he told him its value. "On a really bad day, this blanket would be worth 350,000 dollars and on a good day a half-million dollars." Ted was stunned! If Kit Carson owned it, he said its value would increase by 20%. Ted then became so emotional that he began to gasp for air. He was flabbergasted, knowing his grandparents were just poor farmers. Some of his last words were, "Thank you!" Almost a half-million views have been recorded of this episode on YouTube. Some comments are, "This one really pulls on the heartstrings," or "his reaction is priceless! Congratulations, Sir!"

The blanket was just lying at Ted's home. We have something more valuable than rubies lying at home! What is it? Wisdom, God's word! *"Blessed are those who find wisdom, those who gain understanding.... She is more precious than rubies; nothing you desire can compare with her"* (Proverbs 3:13-15). The good news is we can use it! *"Through wisdom your days will be many, and years will be added to your life. If you are wise, your wisdom will reward you"* (Proverbs 9:11-12). This is a priceless resource that God is providing for our use! *"Trust in the LORD with all your heart and lean not on your own understanding; in all your ways acknowledge him, and he will make your paths straight"* (Proverbs 3:5-6). "Trust" is a concept that includes the idea of safety, confidence, and security. Following God's wisdom creates a sense of security and safety. His wisdom makes life straight, bringing safety, security, confidence, and better health. Learning to acknowledge God and his wisdom in a wide variety of different situations gives us hope. We have something more valuable than rubies or a Navajo Ute chief's blanket!

Watch: at "Top Finds: Mid-19th Century Navajo Ute First Phase Blanket" **https://www.youtube.com/ watch?v=WJw2qCnhea0**

So, to have a good day, use the 17 "Way of Wisdom" principles to outsmart diabetes. Remember these proverbs from God *"are life to those who find them and **health to one's whole body"*** (Proverbs 4:22).

**"The Road to Good Health Is Always Under Construction.
When You Are Through Learning, You Are Through.
Keep Learning!"**

---

*"Those who cherish understanding will
soon prosper"* (Proverbs 19:8).

*"The heart of the discerning acquires knowledge; the
ears of the wise seek it out"* (Proverbs 18:15).

*"A wise man has great power. A man who has knowledge
increases his strength"* (Proverbs 24:5 NIrV).

Many things occupy our time. We may be doing those things right, but are they the things that will contribute to our well-being? If you've read this far, you must be among the discerning who will cherish understanding and prosper. The following story will illustrate **the importance of the 17 wise ways to outsmart diabetes. They are more important than doing things right; they are doing the right things!** Daily doing them brings safety in managing and outsmarting diabetes like this example that illustrates essentials.

Safety

"The wicked flee though no one pursues, but the righteous are as bold as a lion" (Proverbs 28:1). We see a contrast pictured in this verse. Some are afraid and fleeing or fearing being caught without any sense of security. The others, who are righteous, are secure, safe, and confident and are described as being as bold as a lion.

A sense of security is essential, as evidenced by what happened to a hang glider. On his first day of vacation in Switzerland, one person wanted to see the picturesque scenery. Hang gliding off a 4,000-foot ledge was his idea for doing so. Since he had never hang-glided, he hired a pilot. Stepping off the ledge, he realized the pilot had made a critical error—double-checking his safety harness to make sure it was attached to the glider. Carpenters have a rule—measure twice, cut once. They didn't do that. We can see the terrifying crisis that followed because a camera was attached to the glider. The passenger desperately tried to stay alive as he quickly grabbed the pilot's side. He hung onto his side, then reached for the gliding bar with his left hand. The pilot maneuvers the glider with one hand as he holds onto his passenger with his left hand. He eventually puts his left hand on his passenger's left hand for more support.

After one hundred thirty-four seconds of frightening terror, he lets go. By then, they were so close to the ground he landed and only broke his wrist. When he first looked down over a hundred seconds before, he knew this was it—he wouldn't survive. He kept his grip with all his might, not realizing how hard he gripped until later discovering he had torn his left bicep.[83]

People want security and safety in life, which builds their confidence. So many people, however, are going through life like the man whose harness was unattached. They experience one crisis after another. Remember where we started with people fleeing and the others being as bold as a lion? The Hebrew word for "Bold" is often translated as trust and means safety, security, and confidence. The word is used ten times in the Proverbs. Another passage tells us how to have this boldness and confidence. This passage teaches how to have a safety harness attached for security in this life. The teaching is to practice wisdom; by doing so, we trust in God. *"Whoever gives heed to instruction prospers, and blessed is the one who **trusts** in the LORD"* (Proverbs 16:20).

Let's heed planning and careful consideration of what we do: *"The simple believe anything, but the prudent give thought to their steps...The plans of the diligent lead to profit as surely as haste leads to poverty"* (Proverbs 14:15, 21:5). He says he will hang glide again because he "did not get to enjoy my first flight." What do you think will happen with his safety harness?

Watch: "SWISS MISHAP" at **https://www.youtube.com/watch?v=dLBJA8SlH2w&t=163s**

CHAPTER SIX

Practice the Essentials

Additional information on # 1 Keep learning (control the hidden factor of stress on blood glucose levels) and # 2 Have a health routine—a plan with patience, perseverance.

I've read, "You cannot underestimate the unimportance of practically everything." Or "Things which matter most must never be put at the mercy of things which matter least." So many people's lives are cluttered with trivial things that contribute nothing to health and well-being. The 17 wise ways we just examined are the vital few, the essentials for outsmarting diabetes. My brother, a former mathematics professor, says, "17 as a prime number is one of the basic building blocks of whole numbers in mathematics." So, also, are these 17 guidelines basic building blocks for outsmarting diabetes and living well? Using these 17 wise ways for over thirty years, I've maintained an A1c of 5.9–6.4 with only a few exceptions (like my worst result of 7.1 once). I only mention this to let you know how beneficial and effective these wise "common sense" guidelines are.

What should your blood glucose average be? One hundred forty or less, which is an A1c of 6.5 percent or less, according to the American Association of Clinical Endocrinologists; or 7.0

percent or less is what it should be, according to the American Diabetes Association, which is 154 average. A normal A1c is considered 5.6 percent or less.

There is also a concept called the 80/20 principle that has validity. It is the idea that about 80 percent of results come from 20 percent of our actions. We had a peach seedling sprout up in the ground. We put it in a pot and nurtured it until it became big enough to plant in the yard. So, we planted this tiny tree in good soil and watered it occasionally. This nurturing continued after each winter for four years until, in the fifth year, we had a peach tree overflowing with branches burdened with lush, delicious peaches. From a tiny tree, only a few actions brought about more peaches than we can eat. This concept of just a few actions resulting in an abundant harvest Proverbs 27:23-27 explains with an agricultural picture for life or a metaphor for wise management. (*"For they*—teachings for skillful liv-ing—*are life to those who find them and health to one's whole body"* Proverbs 4:22.)

"Be sure you know the condition of your flocks; give careful attention to your herds." When we do this, what benefits do we see? Few of us have flocks or herds, but we all have a body that we need to manage for health with a proper lifestyle. A motivat-ing reason is stated: *"for riches do not endure forever, and a crown is not secure for all generations."* Work is necessary to have the income to live. Stress is elevated by this income, resulting in an unhealthy situation for the mind and body.

Beautiful benefits accrue if knowing and careful attention is given daily to work or our health. *"When the hay is removed, and new growth appears, and the grass from the hills is gathered in, the lambs will provide you with clothing and the goats with the price of a field. You will have plenty of goats' milk to feed your family"* (Proverbs 27:23-27).

Stress

Here is an essential factor to know and give careful attention to: stress. Don't forget the harmful effects of stress because stress directly affects our blood glucose levels. Sometimes circumstances present themselves where a person doesn't even feel stressed, but an elevated blood glucose check reveals stress. Stress is the answer for high blood glucose in certain situations. There are other times when one feels stressed. Some of the acute stress symptoms are a pounding heart, rapid pulse, trembling, shaky, dry throat and mouth, change in blood sugar level, sweating, diarrhea, frequent urination, indigestion, and tension headaches. Some of the signs and symptoms of chronic stress are general irritability, easily fatigued, depression, loss of appetite, anxiety, nervousness, chronic muscle pains, and insomnia.[84]

Stress is an ever-present part of life, but we need to control it. Checking blood pressure at the doctor's office often reveals tension. This is called whitecoat hypertension and occurs because of anxiety in the situation, resulting in an elevated blood pressure reading. A few minutes later, checking the blood pressure results in a lower reading because of less tension. When we perceive something as a threat or stressful, the brain recognizes the danger, like a conflict with someone. It releases an array of stress hormones like cortisol, epinephrine (adrenaline), and norepinephrine.[85]

I had a stressful experience at Silver Dollar City while riding the "Giant Barn Swing." Weak was how I felt two hours after eating lunch. So, before getting on the swing, I checked my blood glucose. My feelings were wrong. I was 162 mg/dl. Since I wasn't weak, I rode the swing with my sons. After the two-minute ride, I still felt like my blood sugar was low. This time it was 197 mg/dl (this was before continuous glucose monitors were available). My rapid increase in blood glucose was a result of stress! With elevated levels of the stress hormone cortisol, insulin is less effective. Thus, the result is higher blood glucose levels. To see what I experienced, watch the "Giant Barn Swing at Silver Dollar City" at **https://www.youtube.com/watch?v=irXWWlrKXwk**

How can the way of wisdom help in stressful situations? Practicing wisdom will result in a more peaceful, composed lifestyle. *"My child, do not forget my teaching, but let your heart keep my commandments; for length of days and years of life and abundant welfare they will give you"* (Proverbs 3:1–2 NRS). Another Bible translation puts it the following way: *"My son, do not forget my teaching, but keep my commands in your heart, for they will prolong your life many years and bring you peace and prosperity."*

Several benefits stand out in this reading: a longer life, peace, and abundant welfare. In this case, the word *peace* can mean completeness or wholeness, and *prosperity* can mean abundant well-being. When a person puts this wisdom into practice, like the father instructs his son to do, peace and prosperity can result. This peace will be with God, a calming peace within oneself and in relationships with others. Conflict with others contributes to stress, which can directly affect blood glucose control and, thus, diabetes management and elevated blood pressure! Worry is another stress factor so practice this guidance from Jesus. Jesus teaches us to live life--one day at a time. He says, *"Therefore, do not worry about tomorrow for tomorrow will worry about itself. Each day has enough trouble of its own"* (Matthew 6:34). Living one day at a time, not month or year, is the way to live, have peace, and win over worry and stress!

The following true stories in the news and from the history of diabetes management will show how effective these wise ways are for success in dealing with diabetes, other chronic diseases, or any stressful challenge you may face in life. These wise "common sense" principles in these uplifting, true stories will reinforce their use in your life. Some of their benefits don't happen overnight. They accumulate one-day-at-time with weeks, months, and years of use. That is why I'm giving examples of patience, perseverance, and planning in the following stories.

Great Understanding

An officer couldn't believe the nerve of a pedestrian walking down the highway at a snail's pace at one mile per hour. The pedestrian had no business even being on the highway. He must have been a hundred years old. The officer even talked to him, but the guy just snapped back at him. This officer was not going to leave him alone on the highway. Therefore, he escorted him until he exited the road. Who was this pedestrian? A tortoise![86]

"Annoyingly frustrated" is a good description of people stuck behind a slow highway driver. At such times, everyone needs the great virtue of patience. Paul placed patience as the first virtue he lists as an attribute of love. *"Love is patient; love is kind"* (1 Corinthians 13:4).

Proverbs 14:29 states, *"Whoever is patient has great understanding, but one who is quick-tempered displays folly."* Jumping to conclusions would have been easy to do with the highway walker, but we read to the end of the story with some patience. Then we don't have to assume; we understand that the walker was a tortoise. If we give ourselves time to be patient, we can have a greater understanding. We begin to see the whole picture.

Have a health routine—a plan.
Patience: Giving your plan time to work.

"Whoever is patient has great understanding, but one who is quick-tempered displays folly." (Proverbs 14:29)

Anger (or being quick-tempered) excludes different possibilities and positive results. Folly results from having a "short-fuse" with no time allotted for better choices, seeing things differently, and understanding better. *"Blessed are those who find wisdom, those who gain understanding"* (Proverbs 3:13). Solomon described what understanding brings—long life with honor, value, pleasant ways, peace, and happy life. *"With patience you can convince a ruler, and a gentle word can get through to the hard-headed"* (Proverbs 25:15). Through patience, you gain great understanding and persuade people. Patience means not giving up but continuing to try! Patience is so important, for through patience, you can convince people. How much time should you give to a difficult situation?

Adversity and the Power of Optimism

What would you do if a tree fell on you, pinning you to the ground? The tree trunk is on your legs, breaking your legs. You are experiencing excruciating pain. There is no one near enough to hear your calls for help. You didn't even bring your phone with you to phone for help. Is this a situation of hopelessness? Will you give up or try to endure, not knowing if anyone will ever come looking for you?

I've just described a situation that happened to a man named Jonathan outside his home in Minnesota.[87] He is cutting down some trees on a Thursday, and one of the tree trunks falls on his legs, pinning him to the ground. He's a teacher of English in high school, and in-class teaching begins on Monday. The first day of school is important, and when he doesn't even show up, he's called. He lives by himself, so his family is informed. They look for him and find him. They immediately call the fire department, and it takes them two hours to lift the log off him. Asking him how long he's been pinned, without hesitation, he says, "one hundred hours."

How did he know his ordeal had lasted one hundred hours? He knew because keeping track of time was part of his strategy to endure. He persevered by trying to live for one hour at a time and breaking that hour into five-minute segments. He celebrated with small victories every five minutes. Every five minutes brought success, giving him hope. Meditating, praying, and inventing rhythms were ways of distracting himself from his situation. By doing this, he didn't panic. The county Sheriff's Chief Deputy said, "He had the will to live, and he wasn't ready to go. I don't know many people who could survive an ordeal like that."[88]

This example illustrates the truth of Proverbs 18:14. *"The will to live can get you through sickness, but no one can live with a broken spirit."* If we are ever in a difficult situation, we can break up adversity into small compartments following the principle Jesus gives of taking life one day at a time, not four days or a month or year. *"Do not worry about tomorrow, for tomorrow will worry about itself. Each day has enough trouble of its own"* (Matthew 6:34). Here is another way the principle is put—"Inch by inch, life's a cinch. Yard by yard, life's hard." Jonathan will have a long road to recovery, but he should recover with the attitude he has. *"A man's spirit will sustain him in sickness, But a crushed spirit who can bear?"* (Proverbs 18:14)

Consider that giving time to concerns like diabetes management brings understanding; as in the following cases, it brings life itself. The following three stories concerning two thirteen-year-old teenagers and one fourteen-year-old demonstrate the importance of patience and not giving up.

I told the story in my book "The Way of Wisdom for Diabetes" about the first American who received insulin after Frederick Banting and Charles Best discovered insulin in 1921. His name was James Havens.

The Story of James Havens:
The First American to Receive Insulin

It was about Thanksgiving, 1914 when James Havens was diagnosed with what we today call Type 1 diabetes. He was almost fifteen years old. From that day on, the wisdom principle of planning ahead was intensely used for him. During the next seven-and-a-half years planning was necessary to just keep him alive. He continued to plan the next thirty-eight years until he died, not of diabetes, but colon cancer! The idea of planning, of deciding ahead of time what to do, was followed by his mother, for she meticulously planned his meals, weighing every morsel of food he ate.

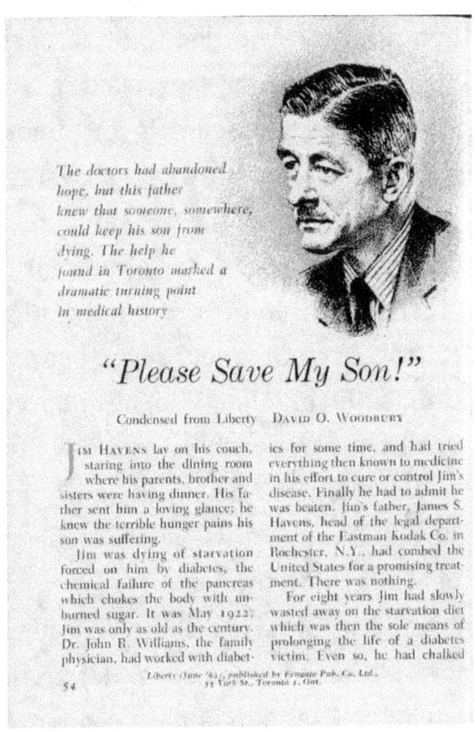

"Please Save My Son!"

Condensed from Liberty   DAVID O. WOODBURY

JIM HAVENS lay on his couch, staring into the dining room where his parents, brother and sisters were having dinner. His father sent him a loving glance; he knew the terrible hunger pains his son was suffering.

Jim was dying of starvation forced on him by diabetes, the chemical failure of the pancreas which chokes the body with unburned sugar. It was May 1922. Jim was only as old as the century. Dr. John R. Williams, the family physician, had worked with diabet-ics for some time, and had tried everything then known to medicine in his effort to cure or control Jim's disease. Finally he had to admit he was beaten. Jim's father, James S. Havens, head of the legal department of the Eastman Kodak Co. in Rochester, N.Y., had combed the United States for a promising treatment. There was nothing.

For eight years Jim had slowly wasted away on the starvation diet which was then the sole means of prolonging the life of a diabetes victim. Even so, he had chalked

Liberty (June '62), published by Fengate Pub. Co. Ltd.,
55 York St., Toronto 1, Ont.

54

A 1963 Reader's Digest condensed story about James Havens, the first American to receive insulin. Photo courtesy of The Thomas Fisher Rare Book Library, University of Toronto.

The subtitle to the Reader's Digest article reads "The doctors had abandoned hope, but this father knew that someone, somewhere, could keep his son from dying. The help he found in Toronto marked a dramatic turning point in medical history."

He was a very fortunate person, as he became the first American to receive insulin. Before insulin, the only therapy was Dr. Frederick Allen's "under-nutrition therapy." Dr. Allen advocated serious dieting to patients, whose complaints were their extreme hunger and rapid weight loss. The doctor seemed to be telling them that they needed to be hungry more often to keep blood sugar levels from skyrocketing higher, eventually leading to coma. Jim endured this for almost eight years until he received insulin. Insulin was discovered in the summer of 1921.

When Jim was diagnosed, he was almost fifteen years old and weighed ninety-seven pounds. From Thanksgiving, 1914, to May 21, 1922, he went from ninety-seven pounds to less than seventy-four pounds. During that time, he endured a meal plan of about 820 calories per day, with painstaking efforts to eliminate most carbohydrates from his meal plan.[89] Deciding ahead of time was required. By doing this, he lived longer than anyone else on this "under-nutrition therapy."

His dad looked and inquired about any new treatments; treatments that would keep his son alive. He was the head of the legal department at the Eastman Kodak Company in Rochester, New York. He searched the United States for eight years, looking for a promising treatment, but none was found. In fact, in March of 1921, his father wrote, "His condition is not such as to hold out any hope."[90]

One day George Snowball, a manager of the Kodak store in Toronto, Canada, came into his office. Mr. Havens asked if he knew anyone in Canada who was working on a cure for diabetes.

He didn't, but he would inquire when he got back home. This man began to ask and ask and eventually discovered that Dr. Banting and his assistant, Charles Best, had made an important discovery at the University of Toronto. Of course, it was *insulin*. When Jim's dad received this exciting news, he persuaded his son's doctor, John Williams, to go to Toronto. While there, Williams was able to get some insulin from Dr. Banting. By May 1922, the only thing Jim could do was moan with excruciating pain. He was barely able to lift his head from his pillow.

He was ready for his life to end. In fact, on his hospital chart, it was recorded that he was "anxious to die and end his misery." He could bear it no longer. Over the next few days, his whole outlook was in for a dramatic change. Dr. Williams was able to bring to Rochester a small amount of unrefined insulin. On the evening of May 21, injections of insulin were started, but they seemed to have no affect.

The next week, George Snowball stopped in to see Jim's dad at Eastman Kodak. When he asked about how Jim was doing, he was surprised to hear his dad say, "I guess we're through." "But those fellows have saved lives," Snowball said.[91] Suddenly Mr. Havens shot up out of his seat and said, "George, get one of those young men over here." Mr. Snowball went to Dr. Banting and pleaded with him to go to New York, but he refused. He refused until Snowball said, "The Havens' physician tried your preparation, and it didn't work. They think it's just another failure."

Dr. Banting went to Rochester, and this time Jim received larger doses of insulin. They gave them in two-hour intervals, checking the urine for sugar at each interval. Eventually, after several doses, they all had a euphoric reaction—no sugar was in the urine. The insulin was working! James wrote to Dr. Banting, the discoverer of insulin: "A week ago last Thursday....Marked an historical event as I then tasted my first egg and toast. Egg on toast is my idea of the only food necessary in heaven."

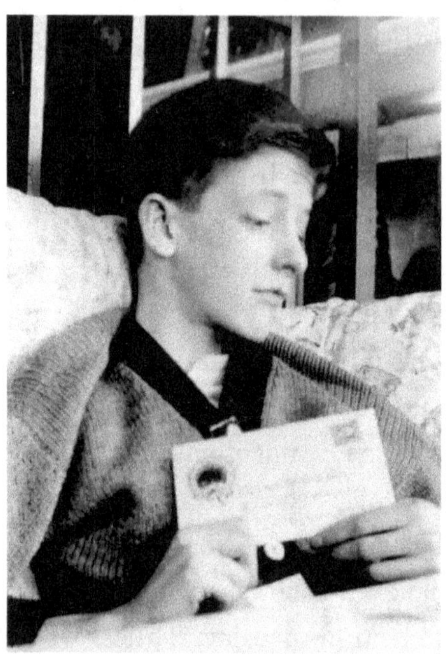

James D. Havens, the first American to receive insulin about 1921. Photo courtesy of The Thomas Fisher Rare Book Library, University of Toronto.

"A cheerful look brings joy to your heart. And good news gives health to your body" (Proverbs 15:30 NIrV). We can be thankful today that we don't have to endure what James Havens had to face. His comment after receiving insulin was a comment of gratitude! When I realize we have so many new resources available today like glucose meters, new types of insulin, insulin

pumps and pens, and an assortment of medications, and other ways to prevent or cope with complications that weren't available more than fifty years ago, I am overwhelmed with gratitude! I believe this gratitude perspective can help anyone face the challenge to outsmart diabetes when used daily.

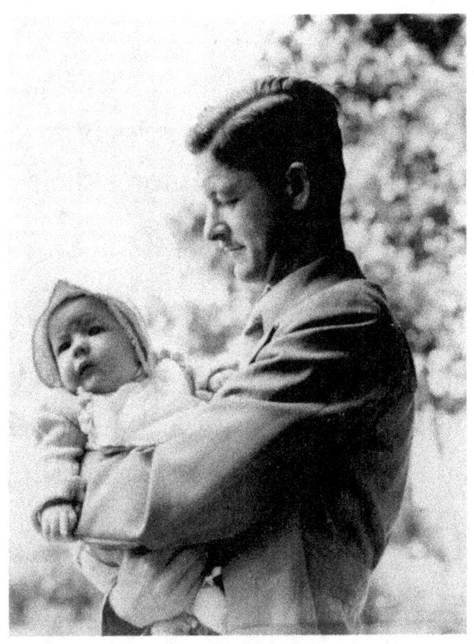

James Havens holding one of his children. He died in 1960, but not of diabetes complications but of colon cancer. Photo courtesy of The Thomas Fisher Rare Book Library, University of Toronto.

For more than seven years, James Havens persevered with the support of his parents. With patience and perseverance, his life was saved. He continued to plan his meals and take daily injections of insulin for the rest of his life. If he hadn't been one of the fortunate ones at that time his life would have been over. Instead, he lived another thirty-eight years, got married and had a family. We never know what wonderful results will appear when we persevere with patience and planning. We too have access to these powerful principles of planning, perseverance, and patience. *"Do not those who plot evil go astray? But those who plan what is good find love and faithfulness...Sluggards do not plow in season; so at harvest time they look but find nothing...The plans of the diligent lead to profit as surely as haste leads to poverty"* (Proverbs 14:22, 20:4, 21:5). As a result, we'll be rewarded for using them, which will then reinforce their repeated use in our lives.

A Freak Accident

Thirteen-year-old Trenton was in a freak accident. His friend was driving a utility vehicle and pulling him in an attached wagon. He came around a corner too fast and flipped the wagon. Trenton's head hit the ground, and the wagon landed on his head, causing seven skull fractures. After being rushed to the hospital, a doctor admitted he had "no brain waves, a damaged brain stem, and his heart only beat because of adrenaline." He was in a coma and on life support in the hospital. If he were to regain consciousness, he would be like a vegetable.

His future looked bleak. After weeks in this condition, his parents signed papers to donate Trenton's organs to five children. The day before his doctors scheduled his life support to end, he moved his fingers and then a foot and regained consciousness. Soon Trenton was shooting baskets from his wheelchair in the hospital gym. His mom said he is healing daily; she praises the Lord for his recovery. He has his full memory. He talks about his school friends. His healing continues now at home.[92]

Have you ever heard anyone answer "how are you" with "hanging in there?" I usually say, "don't let go." God's wisdom says, *"Whoever is patient has great understanding"* (Proverbs 14:29). Keep hanging on with patience because patience gives an understanding that healing takes time. Have you ever done physical therapy for weeks with no results, and then suddenly, the treatment begins to work? If you ever need patience under challenging circumstances, remember Proverbs 14:29! Just quote it. You will be surprised at how helpful the repeating of God's wisdom is.

Watch: Miracle Boy' Trenton McKinley Wakes From Coma Just Before Organ Harvesting | TODAY at **https://www.youtube.com/watch?v=Krpdx6YyCTA**

"Love is patient. Love is kind" (1 Corinthians 13:4)

Here is another example of patience and an optimistic attitude.

783 Days

A recent human-interest story concerned a thirteen-year-old girl who needed a heart transplant. After being on the transplant list for 783 days, she was scheduled to get a pacemaker, not a heart. They had not found an available heart, and her health had worsened so that she couldn't wait any longer. Anna's zest for life, her desire, and her optimism were never a concern; instead, it was the problem with her heart.

The transplant team had scheduled her to be at Texas Children's Hospital at six in the morning, and her mother said, "They were short on beds." She was beginning to wonder if it was even going to happen. Four hours later, nurses were finally prepping Anna for her surgery. Anna even got the IV. But then there was more waiting. The family wondered if they had gone to lunch and forgotten about Anna. They sat for another hour and a half. Finally, Anna's transplant coordinator entered the room with several other people. They said, "Anna, are you excited about getting your ICD (implantable cardioverter-defibrillator) today?" She said, "I guess so," and the coordinator said, "How would you like a new heart instead?"

One week after receiving a new heart, she became stronger daily, walking, talking, and smiling. The family concluded that if the initially scheduled surgery had happened on time, the donor heart for which they had waited 783 days would have gone to someone else. The delay saved her that day![93]

God's wisdom is aptly seen in this beautiful story too. How? We see the value of patience, an optimistic attitude, and perseverance all on display! It's evident from this story that patience does carry a lot of wait. Too many people are not willing to wait. She wouldn't have experienced a new heart if she had given up. We can grasp the full meaning of the proverb that *"Those who are patient have great understanding"* (Proverbs 14:29). She could understand the value in staying optimistic, not giving up and waiting day in and day out for 783 days because they are what brought her to the point of receiving a new heart! Her optimistic attitude sustained her through this sickness. *"The will to live can get you through sickness, but no one can live with a broken spirit"*

(Proverbs 18:14 NCV). The temptation is to expect quick results, but the wise thing to do is stay patient and optimistic and trust God and his wisdom. *"Eat honey, my son, for it is good; honey from the comb is sweet to your taste. Know also that wisdom is sweet to your soul; if you find it, there is a future hope for you, and your hope will not be cut off"* (Proverbs 24:13-14).

How to Live with Diabetes When Doctors Diagnosed Me as a Seven-Year-Old in 1960

With all the resources available today, you are now living in the best of times to outsmart diabetes. Add to the resources the principles of God's wisdom, His optimism, like gratitude, patience, perseverance, and discernment, and you can succeed! When I was diagnosed with diabetes in December of 1960, the book "How to Live with Diabetes" by Henry Dolger, M.D. was given to me (Dr. Dolger was the Distinguished Chief of The Medical Staff of the Mount Sinai Diabetes Clinic, New York City). Very little was known about diabetes then compared to what is known today.

There was only one oral medication when this book was written. The medication was called Orinase. Dr. Dolger wrote, "Where the patients were between 20 and 40, Orinase was effective in four out of five cases. In juvenile diabetes and where the patients were under 20, Orinase was rarely effective. Also, he writes, "There is no relation to the length of time a person has had diabetes and his response to Orinase. Long-standing cases showed good response, as did new cases. Nor was the body type of the patient a factor in response to Orinase." He continued, "Clearly, for a large number of diabetics, Orinase presaged a revolution in treatment virtually as great as that brought about by the discovery of insulin."[94] There were several theories given as to why it worked, but the right one was the stimulation of the pancreas to secrete insulin.

Now medications are available that use incretin hormones like Ozempic and Mounjaro (**read more on these medications in Wise Way # 12 and their side effects**), DPP4 enzyme inhibitors, slow down the digestive system, prevent the release of stored glucose or glycogen in the liver and others that help with blood glucose control in the kidneys independent of insulin. There are injectable combinations of these medications that are injected daily or just once a week.

When I was first diagnosed sixty-four+ years ago, only thick hypodermic needles were available. Dr. Dolger wrote, "It should be 25 to 26 gauge (the size gauge used with animals today). A reserve supply of needles should always be kept on hand because needles may bend or break and, in any case, usually become dull after about two weeks' use."[95] I remember those needles becoming dull and very uncomfortable with each painful injection. Today we use insulin pens or syringes with ultra-thin needles with gauges of 31 or 32. Yes, we've come to a much better day for living well. **So, keep working on control with patience, perseverance, and knowledgeable judgment of what to do each day, and you, too, will succeed.**

CHAPTER SEVEN

Stay OPTIMISTIC with Gratitude

Additional information on # 6—Focus on staying OPTIMISTIC every day with gratitude.

Scientific research on gratitude has demonstrated many incredible benefits. Benefits include being more optimistic, connected with others, sleeping better, being more compliant in following a meal and exercise plan, and taking medicine. These benefits also reduce stress, decreasing levels of counter-regulatory hormones like epinephrine (adrenaline) and cortisol that cause insulin resistance and elevated blood glucose. Here are stories that illustrate and reinforce the practice of gratitude.

Positive Focus

"A cheerful heart is good medicine, but a crushed spirit dries up the bones" (Proverbs 17:22). A cheerful heart is good medicine. Laughter, smiles, and even tears came to a family when their baby daughter heard her older sister for the first time after she received hearing aids. The older sister kept saying, "Baby sister, baby sister," and then the baby sister began to giggle and laugh. Laughing and laughing, she started jumping up and down on

her mother's knee as her older sister continued to talk to her. Gasping with joy, the mother covered her mouth. She could not contain her tears of joy. Smiling and looking up at her mom, she pauses and then breaks out with laughter again as she looks at her sister. The whole scene displayed the truth of the proverb that a cheerful heart is good medicine! Why do scenes like that bring joy to all of us? The reason is we like good news. This was certainly good news for the baby and her family! *A cheerful look brings joy to your heart. And good news gives health to your body*" (Proverbs 15:30). When people are diagnosed with diabetes, lifestyle changes need to happen. So, we shouldn't fear change because, as this story illustrates, good news in one's life and well-being can result!

Watch: "Baby Girl Can't Hide Her Happiness at Hearing Her Sister's Voice for the First Time" at **https://www.youtube.com/watch?v=2qPzucf_Yxo**

Here is another beautiful good news story. Standing in a grocery checkout line is often frustrating, especially if yours is just slowly moving. What if you were waiting and then realizing you forgot your billfold? This happened to an older man one day. His frustration and alarm turned into good news, as the person ahead of him was an observant young woman who offered to pay for his groceries. He was very appreciative, wanted to pay her back, and asked for her mailing address. Sure enough, a few days later, she received a fifteen-dollar check with this note. "You saved me a lot of trouble. My wife is ill, and I wanted to get back to her. I'm not very young anymore—84 years old. It's not a surprise I left my wallet at home. I shall always remember your kindness." This was good news for the man and the young woman. She doesn't plan to cash the check. She says, "I have something that I look at every morning when I leave my room. It says 'be the reason that someone smiles today' so I see that when I leave my house. That was what I could do to make him smile that day."[96]

Stories like these build goodwill and gratitude in life. I'm thankful I saw the video and could read the notes from the incident at the grocery store. Positive stories like these are where God's wisdom directs us. *"He who seeks good finds goodwill, but evil comes to him who searches for it"* (Proverbs 11:27).

"If You're Happy and You Know It . . ."

"A happy heart makes the face cheerful, but heartache crushes the spirit...All the days of the oppressed are wretched, but the cheerful heart has a continual feast" (Proverbs 15:13, 15). What contributes to a continuous cheerful feast? We must keep pumping in the air to keep a leaky tire from going flat. To keep a cheerful heart from falling into the gloomy depths of dreariness, we must keep pumping the heart with thoughts from the brighter side of life! Some of these ideas are not only good but can be humorous as well.

For example, let Phoebe, who is a Cockatiel, cheer us. I heard Phoebe chirping the opening tune of "If You're Happy and You Know It." The next phrase is "Clap your hands." Since she has no hands, she uses her beak to tap on a banana or the table to "clap your hands." She enthusiastically continues to do this for over a minute, building up to a final crescendo.

When you click on this link, "Bird Sings If You're Happy and You Know It"at **https://www.youtube.com/watch?v=zFxwNlccSt4,**

Health Applications to a positive, grateful attitude

The study "Diabetes Attitudes, Wishes and Needs" was conducted in 2011 with almost 8600 people with Type 1 and Type 2 Diabetes. The research was done primarily in North America and Europe. The study revealed attitudes that need strengthening and coping with challenging needs.

People answered open-ended questions about impacting experiences, challenges, successes, and wishes for personal improvement. Expressed were the need to not always be on guard and the desire for less anxiety and worry. Fifty-six percent were afraid, and one of the big fears was hypoglycemia (low blood sugar). One elderly woman expressed this fear by saying, "I was living by myself and I had a hypoglycemic crisis. I was no longer able to understand anything; they told me I did not make sense when I talked and that I wasn't able to move, to sleep calmly, to recognize my children."[97] (At the end of this chapter, I will show how I've eliminated fear and successfully dealt with low blood sugar or hypoglycemia for six decades). Forty-five percent hoped for "less anxiety and worry," as in "I wish I didn't have to have my guard up." One woman said, "This illness makes me very afraid, even if I am used to it." Others were afraid they would not be able to control their diabetes.

What caught my attention, too, were people's negative moods—even a sense of hopelessness. One person said, "When everything is going well, I am well, and so is the diabetes. On the other hand, however, whenever I have a bout of the blues or my morale is low, it goes out of whack, and the diabetes is like a yo-yo."[98] Is any of this surprising? No, consider the challenges we all face, whether health issues or other stressful situations. What we need, what we must strive for, is optimism, a positive attitude. It's not just a coping mechanism, it's a powerful tool in managing diabetes and improving the quality of life.

Elizabeth Hughes and the Power of Optimism

The news of a diagnosis of diabetes can be overwhelming. People may begin to worry about doing all the diabetes procedures correctly. They can be upset because they have to make too many changes. Who likes change? They may have to change their eating habits and learn how carbohydrates, exercise, and medications affect blood sugar levels. Creating a routine to manage these changes is essential for checking blood sugar levels, taking medications, and planning meals. By doing this, you will feel more in control and less overwhelmed.

The downward pull of discouragement can occur while thinking negatively about the future. Let's remember what the way of wisdom states about our thinking: *"Be careful what you think, because your thoughts run your life"* (Proverbs 4:23 NCV). Have you ever heard yourself (or others) saying, "I did everything I was supposed to, and my blood glucose readings are still all over the place!" "I tried that new medication, and I don't feel any better." "For two months now, I've been walking regularly, but I haven't lost an ounce of weight!"

What Are You Saying to Yourself about Low Blood Sugars?

Someone may tell the person recently diagnosed with diabetes about low blood sugar or hypoglycemia and imagine how it can feel. It is one thing to think of it intellectually and another to experience it. When the person experiences it, they may be thinking, "This will ruin everything—my ability to drive safely and confidently as well as manage my diabetes successfully," or "Good diabetes care is now impossible. My life will be wrecked." Neither one of those statements is true. People need to learn what to do when low blood sugar occurs—and to talk to themselves more pleasantly and reassuringly.

One of the symptoms of a low blood sugar count, or hypoglycemia, is feeling physically weaker, perhaps not having the energy even to walk. A person can also feel very hungry. If left untreated, blurry vision and incoherency can result. Hypoglycemia is a 70 mg/dl reading or less. How many grams of quick-energy carbohydrates are needed to treat a low blood glucose reading? A good rule of thumb is that 1 gram of glucose raises the blood sugar 3, 4, or 5 points for body weights of 200, 150, or 100 pounds, respectively. For example, 5 grams of dextrose, as found in Smarties® or SweeTarts®, raises the blood sugar by about 20 points for a 150-lb person. **More on coping with hypoglycemia in Wise Way # 16—Correct low-blood glucose: hypoglycemia.**

It Is Nice to Have Support

In these situations, it would be good to have a support system. As a supporter, it's good to understand how it feels to experience a 255 mg/dl high blood glucose or a 55 mg/dl low. Listen to how those with diabetes describe the highs and lows at "Highs and Lows" **https://www.youtube.com/watch?v=zKVT5GB dVK8&list=PL72C20AB88463B658&index=22** Sometimes people are overwhelmed with good support, whereas others are virtually on their own. The following two illustrations show the stark contrast.

One night, a couple who had been married for over fifty years was lying in bed. The husband was almost asleep when he heard his wife sobbing, and he asked, "Honey, what's wrong?" "There was a time when you would give me a good night kiss before going to sleep," she said. He then kissed her. He was about asleep again when his wife began to cry. "What's wrong, honey?" "There was a time when you would hold my hand before going to sleep." He then held her hand. She began to cry again when he was almost asleep. "Honey, what's wrong?" "There was a time when you would nibble on my ear before going to sleep." With that, he got right up out of bed. She said, "Honey, don't be mad, don't be mad!" He said, "Who's mad? I'm just going to get my teeth."

I like that attitude, don't you? Service can make a tremendous difference, not only to others but also to the one giving it! Wisdom's way teaches, *"Whoever refreshes others will be refreshed"* (Proverbs 11:25). According to that passage, when we support others with diabetes, we also help and encourage ourselves.

Now, compare that example with the following one. A doctor is talking to the patient's wife and says, "Madam, unless you do the following, your husband isn't going to be around too long." The doctor gave this prescription: "Make sure he gets a good, healthy breakfast every morning. "Have him come home for lunch daily so you can feed him a low-fat, high-fiber, balanced meal. Make sure you serve him a hot supper every night, and don't burden him with any household chores." "Also," the doctor continued, "Keep the house spotless, so he's never exposed to any unnecessary germs." Later, on the way home, the husband asked his wife what the doctor had said. She paused momentarily and said, "Honey, the doctor thinks you won't be around too much longer!"

The Best Support of All

There is a glaring contrast in those two situations, isn't there? Some have very supportive people, while others aren't so fortunate! What we overlooked in both of the examples is where we can find the best support. Dr. Gary Arsham, a Type 1 Diabetic, puts it this way: "You are the best available source of support for living well with diabetes. You are always there and you know yourself well. No one else can take care of you as well as you can."[99]

For example, the way of wisdom states: *"The wise in heart are called discerning, and gracious (pleasant) words promote instruction"* (Proverbs 16:21). Not only can pleasant words promote instruction with others, but they can also promote instruction when we use them with ourselves! *"For as he thinks within himself, so he is"* (Proverbs 23:7 NAS). We can use positive thinking to our advantage! *"A tongue that brings healing is like a tree of life. But a tongue that tells lies produces a broken spirit"* (Proverbs 15:4 NIrV). We can even deceive ourselves about our future and be crushed and not healed. Instead of feeling guilty or ashamed for having diabetes, being anxious about learning all the things necessary to live well, or fearing complications, why not talk to ourselves with pleasant, encouraging words? *"Pleasant words are like honey. They are sweet to the spirit and bring healing to the body"* (Proverbs 16:24 NIrV).

"Things turn out best for those who make the best out of the way that things turn out." Making the best decisions out of tragedy was profoundly demonstrated in a sixteen-year-old who survived a shark attack. He lost his left arm while he was waist-deep in water on a beach in North Carolina.

As he is being interviewed in his hospital bed, recovering from the shock of what happened, he says something very profound and wise for a sixteen-year-old. "I have two options: I can try to live my life the way I was and make an effort to do that even though I don't have an arm, or I can just let this be completely debilitating and bring my life down and ruin it," Hunter Treschl said. "Out of those two, there's really only one that I would actually choose and that's to try to fight and live a normal life with the cards I've been dealt." Confronting the challenges and accepting reality is the attitude we all need when facing the challenges of diabetes, too. Watch the interview "North Carolina double shark attack: Teenager Hunter Treschl speaks out about losing arm." at **https://www.youtube.com/watch?v=0uJkkVZW_FI** .

Elizabeth Hughes was diagnosed with diabetes at the age of eleven and spent the next four years on the "under-nutrition, starvation therapy" prescribed by Dr. Frederick Allen. We can be thankful that we don't have to go through what she experienced. We can also see, however, essential characteristics Elizabeth had that we should emulate. It was her focus on good things in challenging circumstances that helped her to live through the pain and hunger she faced. She used pleasant words and gratitude principles in her letters to her mother.

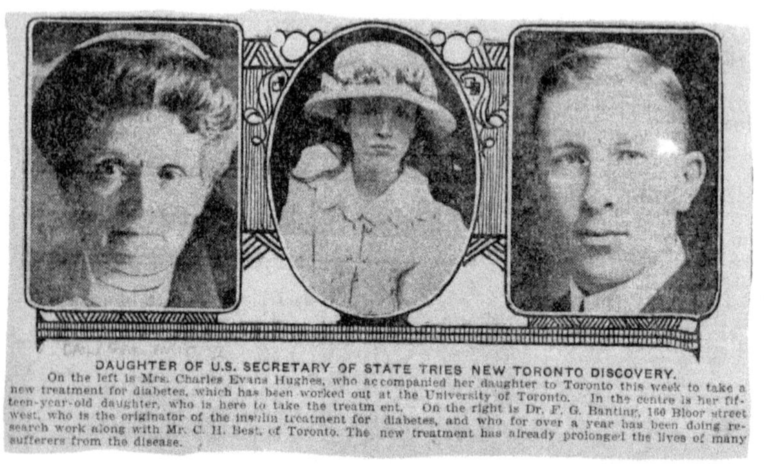

DAUGHTER OF U.S. SECRETARY OF STATE TRIES NEW TORONTO DISCOVERY.
On the left is Mrs. Charles Evans Hughes, who accompanied her daughter to Toronto this week to take a new treatment for diabetes, which has been worked out at the University of Toronto. In the centre is her fifteen-year-old daughter, who is here to take the treatment. On the right is Dr. F. G. Banting, 160 Bloor street west, who is the originator of the insulin treatment for diabetes, and who for over a year has been doing research work along with Mr. C. H. Best, of Toronto. The new treatment has already prolonged the lives of many sufferers from the disease.

Elizabeth Hughes, daughter of U.S. Secretary of State tries new Toronto discovery August 17, 1922. Photo courtesy of the Thomas Fisher Rare Book Library, University of Toronto.

Economic status did not exempt people from being diagnosed with diabetes then, just as it doesn't now. Her father, Charles Hughes, had been the governor of New York; he went on to hold various offices, such as the United States Secretary of State under the Harding administration and later a Supreme Court Justice. When doctors diagnosed her with diabetes in 1918, at the age of eleven, she was five feet tall and weighed seventy-five pounds. When Dr. Frederick Banting, the discoverer of insulin, examined her on August 16, 1922, three days before her fifteenth birthday, she weighed forty-five pounds.

After being diagnosed, her parents could afford to hire a nurse, Blanche Burgess, to help her. Dr. Elliott Joslin of Boston had trained her. Ultimately, however, as was previously mentioned, the best available source of support for managing diabetes is from the one who has it. She would have to learn and adhere to what was required to live. She had learned self-control and discipline from her parents, which helped her tremendously.

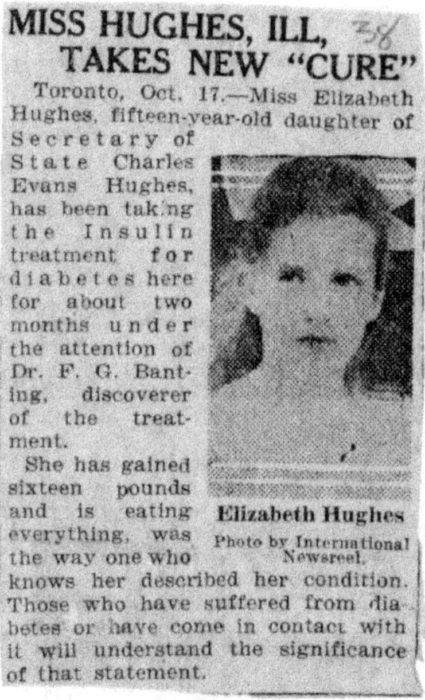

MISS HUGHES, ILL, TAKES NEW "CURE"

Toronto, Oct. 17.—Miss Elizabeth Hughes, fifteen-year-old daughter of Secretary of State Charles Evans Hughes, has been taking the Insulin treatment for diabetes here for about two months under the attention of Dr. F. G. Banting, discoverer of the treatment.

She has gained sixteen pounds and is eating everything, was the way one who knows her described her condition. Those who have suffered from diabetes or have come in contact with it will understand the significance of that statement.

Elizabeth Hughes

Photo by International Newsreel.

Miss Hughes, ill, takes new "cure." Photo courtesy of the Thomas Fisher Rare Book Library, University of Toronto.

The way of wisdom states: *"Like a city whose walls are broken through is a person who lacks self-control"* (Proverbs 25:28). A defense mechanism for cities in ancient times was their walls, which protected them from enemy armies. The wise state that our defense is self-control, which can be used against onslaughts of overeating delicious food, sitting too much, or just giving up on following a healthy plan. It is interesting how Elizabeth's focus reinforced her self-control, as she wrote in her letters to her mother.

There were times during the next four years, after being diagnosed with diabetes, that she consumed as little as four hundred calories per day. By the spring of 1921, she only weighed fifty-two pounds. She could only eat a mundane diet of food that kept her from showing sugar in her urine. Her father was the Secretary of State, and their home was in Washington, DC. In that environment of political stress, she could not attain proper control.

They could not keep an atmosphere of peace and calm for her; there was just too much activity. Her parents decided to send her to the island of Bermuda for six months, accompanied by her nurse.

She loved to write to her mother during her stay, and what she decided to write about was interesting. She could have written about her intense sense of hunger and weakness, but there would be little new to say about that. Instead, her letters were an upbeat recounting of her days. After researching her letters, Catherine Cox wrote, "She might have been writing cheerful letters because that was what she wanted to receive.... She kept her letters focused on the positive and downplayed the inconveniences of her condition....It is also possible that with her upbeat tone she was just trying to think positively." [100] Of course, Elizabeth Hughes was one of the fortunate ones to receive some of the first insulin doses. She described it as, "Oh, it is simply too wonderful for words this stuff."[101] She died in 1981 after taking at least 42,000 injections of insulin over fifty-eight years!

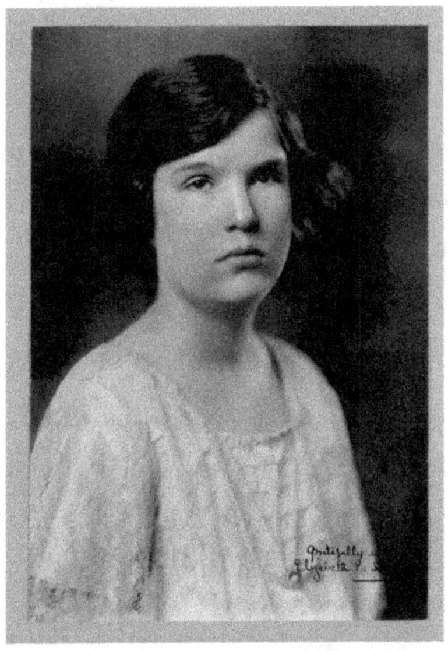

Elizabeth Hughes after receiving insulin, about 1923.
Photo courtesy of the Thomas Fisher Rare Book
Library, University of Toronto.

Choose the Color

A sympathetic friend said to a disabled woman, "Affliction does so color life." "Yes," the woman replied, "but I propose to choose the color." Isn't that what Elizabeth did? She chose her attitude. The way of wisdom states: *"The will to live can get you through sickness, but no one can live with a broken spirit,"* (NCV) or, translated differently, *"The spirit of a man will sustain him in sickness, But who can bear a broken spirit?"* (Proverbs 18:14 NKJV).

When the apostle Paul was in prison, he wrote this advice to the Philippians: *"Finally, my brothers and sisters, always think about what is true. Think about what is noble, right and pure. Think about what is lovely and worthy of respect. If anything is excellent or worthy of praise, think about those kinds of things"* (Philippians 4:8). He points out that we can choose how we think. This is God's way of wisdom. Endurance and better health come by focusing on the good news! *"A cheerful look brings joy to your heart. And good news gives health to your body"* (Proverbs 15:30 NIrV).

In summary, have great expectations of yourself. Realize what advantages you have available today. Remember these three phrases from God's wisdom the way of wisdom: *"Pleasant words are like honey. They are sweet to the spirit and bring healing to the body"* (Proverbs 16:24 NIrV), and *"If you are wise; your wisdom will reward you"* (Proverbs 9:12). Live a life of gratitude and express your thanks as these stories reveal.

Stay Fresh and Green

Another encouraging story is the story of Dr. Robert Moore. This San Jose man's 100th birthday celebration went to the dogs last Saturday. Literally! The family decided to honor their father, who loves dogs and is known as a dog whisperer, by having a parade of dogs in front of his house so he could pet them. Those who wanted to wish him happy birthday were to come with their dogs dressed in cowboy hats, or tuxedos, and so on. They put the notice on the Nextdoor app expecting maybe twenty to thirty dogs. To their surprise, more than two hundred dogs came! The line extended around the block and down the street, for there were so many. There were pups with disabilities, dogs pulling carts, and even canines in classic cars. Dr. Robert Moore, former dean at San Jose State University, with his avid love of dogs, demonstrated it that day by petting each one who came and thanking the owners of each dog!

The Moore family was heartened by how the community came with their dogs and brought him flowers, cupcakes, drawings, and posters. His daughter said, "My father, he was so touched. He pet every single dog that came through. Every person brought the dog up to him. It was so lovely." Yes, even at 100, I see his fresh and green attitude, as the psalmist expressed. *"The righteous will flourish like a palm tree, they will grow like a cedar of Lebanon; planted in the house of the LORD, they will flourish in the courts of our God. They will still bear fruit in old age, they will stay fresh and green, proclaiming, 'The LORD is upright; he is my Rock, and there is no wickedness in him'"* (Psalm 92:12-15). Let's all strive to have that attitude each day!

Focusing on stories like this is the practice of **God's wisdom.** *"He who seeks good finds goodwill, but evil comes to him who searches for it"* (Proverbs 11:27). It is meaningful that Proverbs 17:22 states, *"a cheerful heart is good medicine."* By reading these stories and watching Phoebe, the Cockatiel, we will experience the good medicine that brings a cheerful heart. *"A cheerful look brings joy to your heart. And good news gives health to your body"* (Proverbs 15:30).

"How good is a timely word" (Proverbs 15:23).

"A word fitly spoken is like apples of gold in a setting of silver" (Proverbs 25:11). One word can make a difference in a person's

life. One word made the difference for a soldier in the Vietnam War almost fifty years ago. What was that word? Was it love, compassion, kindness, or gentleness? No, although it expressed those ideas, "thanks" was the word.

A sixth-grade girl completed her homework assignment with "thanks." She sent a letter of encouragement to a soldier—a soldier she did not even know! John has kept this note ever since he received it for Christmas 1970. Following is the message sent to him: "Dear Serviceman, I want to give my sincere thanks for going over to war to fight for us. The class hopes you will be able to come home."

"Thanks" is a powerful word of appreciation that is sparingly used. Remember when Jesus healed the ten lepers how many came back to him and said thanks? Yes, only one came back and used that word to thank him.

Any soldier could have received the girl's note, but John appreciated it. His job was dangerous on a helicopter each day. He said, "When you got up in the morning, you always wondered whether you would see the sun go down at night." He still has the note hidden behind a picture in his living room.

John's family found DonnaCaye, the sixth-grade girl who wrote the thankful message. They even arranged a surprise meeting. When he saw her, he exclaimed, "You're real." "I'm real," DonnaCaye said, and "I remember writing the letter. I was amazed that I could have the opportunity to write to a serviceman and maybe make his life a little simpler for a couple of minutes." Her word of "thanks" has continued to help past those first minutes. The words have continued to encourage him for almost fifty years. "Fact is, I think it means more today than it did when I got it," John admitted. He received thanks; he still treasures it![102]

Words have power as the proverb says. *"What you say can mean life or death. Those who speak with care will be rewarded"* (Proverbs 18:21 NCV). We see from this note that both were rewarded! The apostle Paul writes, *"and be thankful...give thanks in all circumstances for this is God's will for you in Christ Jesus"* (Colossians 3:15, 1 Thessalonians 5:18).

Expressing Gratitude

An easy way to express gratitude is a simple "Thank You." Sometimes we encounter people who are due a great deal of gratitude. At a restaurant one day, we met a man who deserved a "thank you!" We tried to live out the teachings of Proverbs 3:27-28. ***"Do not withhold good from those who deserve it, when it is in your power to act.*** *Do not say to your neighbor, 'Come back later; I'll give it tomorrow'—when you now have it with you."* Waiting for a table at a busy IHOP, we sat on a cushioned bench in the entry. Seeing an older man with his son enter, we moved over, making room for them. I said with a smile, "We want to respect our elders." He smiled and sat down, and we began to talk. You must be 85! No, I will turn 96 in a couple of months. Well, you look healthy for your age. He then proceeded to tell about a couple of surgeries he recently had. He admitted that he shouldn't have even been around to have such operations.

He was in the World War II battle that everyone has heard about—Iwo Jima. The five-week fight was one of the fiercest battles in the Pacific during World War II. Thousands lost their lives. He was near an ammunition depot when a live shell landed. If it goes off, over a hundred men will die. Solders begin scurrying away while he jumped nearer the shell along with two others. Grabbing the shell and throwing it away from the ammunition, they saved lives. He received a Citation of Honor for saving over a hundred men. We have all seen pictures of the marines lifting "Old Glory" to symbolize their victory. He remembers seeing them raise the flag firsthand.

How often do we hear stories of heroism like that while waiting for a table at a restaurant? We began thinking about how commendable his act of courage and kindness was on that day almost 75 years ago. After hearing about his heroic actions that day at IHOP, the wisdom teaching of Proverbs 3:27 came to our minds. ***"Do not withhold good from those who deserve it, when it is in your power to act."*** In appreciation, we decided to pay for their meal. We inquired, but technology got in the way. The son's smartphone had an IHOP app, and he had already paid. Even though that particular expression of gratitude did not turn out, we can all try to find ways to express gratitude with kindness to others!

"Make sure that nobody pays back wrong for wrong, but always try to be kind to each other and to everyone else." (1 Thessalonians 5:15)

CHAPTER EIGHT

Get Up and Move for Living Well

Additional information on # 7—
Move often throughout Every Day.

If you were told about a once-a-day pill that could help you sleep better, restore your energy, improve your mood, reduce your risk of heart disease, help you to lose weight, and improve your blood sugar control, you would probably take it in an instant! And movement does all of that! It doesn't even stop there, because it can also increase your good cholesterol (HDL), lower your bad cholesterol (LDL), and improve blood pressure. If you have a gloomy mood, then move more. Movement can stimulate the brain to release endorphins, which are positive mood changers, and also release serotonin, which can stave off depression.[103]

Let me give you a practical example of patience (plus perseverance) and movement. After having an MRI on my shoulder, the results came several weeks later. My appointment to see a surgeon was scheduled. I was sure surgery was certain; however, he told me that 80% of people with my shoulder condition can avoid surgery through physical therapy. Happily, I then used two wisdom principles—patience and persistence. I patiently went through six weeks of physical therapy and persistently did the exercises at home. When I saw him again, he tested my strength and flexibility. He proclaimed no surgery is necessary if I continue physical therapy at home. Patience and persistence are so compatible; they work together like a hand in a glove. And that is what we need to use for exercise results—patience and persistence. Let's look at the research about the benefits of movement and some good examples we should emulate.

10,000 Steps or Move More Prescription

Should 10,000 steps per day be our goal? The way of wisdom instructs us to move more. *"Go to the ant, you sluggard; consider its ways and be wise!...Ants are creatures of little strength, yet they store up their food in the summer"* (Proverbs 30:25).

Just think of ants! What are some of their characteristics? They are fast and strong. Ants take the initiative and don't let obstacles stop them. They'll go over, around, or under them so they don't give up. They're persistent! They are always on the move—industrious, moving, saving, storing. In fact, how many couch potato ants have you seen? Of course, moving relates directly to our physical well-being and health.

So, should 10,000 steps per day be our goal? Who came up with the idea to walk 10,000 steps a day? In Japan, people were thinking about fitness during the 1964 Tokyo Olympics. During that time, a Japanese company started selling a pedometer called a "manpo-kei—"man" stands for 10,000, "po" for step, and "kei" for gauge. It was a simple marketing campaign name by a

Japanese company. Doctor Yoshiro Hatano led the campaign's research. He determined the average person took 3,500 to 5,000 steps per day and that if they were to increase their steps to 10,000, the result would be healthier, thinner people!

Can we conclude that the Japanese diet of the 1960s was the same as the calorie-rich diets of Americans today? The number of Americans with diabetes and prediabetes is estimated at one hundred thirty-five million.[104] Are we today as healthy as the Japanese were in the 1960s? Theodore Bestor, a Harvard researcher of Japanese society, says, "By all accounts, life in Japan in the 1960s was less calorie-rich, less animal fat, and much less bound up in cars."[105] What should the number of steps per day be?

A study of Scottish postal workers found that the workers averaged 15,000 steps per day. They were fit with healthy waistlines, cholesterol levels, and a lower risk of heart disease. What is the average number of steps of people per day in the United States? According to new Stanford University research, people in the U.S. only average 4,774 steps daily.[106] Is this a good number? According to the CDC, more than one-third (36.5%) of U.S. adults are obese, which relates to this low number of daily steps.[107]

Amish Study

There would have been no modern technological conveniences in the first century and earlier centuries. People's lifestyles required a greater level of physical activity during those times. In 2004, researchers from the University of Tennessee studied the activity level among ninety-eight participants aged eighteen and seventy-five from an Old Order Amish community in southern Ontario. Their lifestyle requires abstaining from driving automobiles, using electrical appliances, or other modern conveniences. Their way of life has stayed the same for the last one hundred fifty years. Farming is still the predominant occupation. Researchers asked them to wear a pedometer for seven days during June and to fill out a log sheet on which they recorded their number of steps per day and physical activities.

Fifty-three men and forty-five women participated, and they discovered a high level of physical activity. The Amish men reported doing an average of ten hours of vigorous activity and about forty-three hours of moderate activity per week. The women reported doing about three and a half hours of vigorous activity and thirty-nine hours of moderate activity per week. The average number of steps per day was almost stunning! The average number of daily steps was 18,425 for men versus 14,196 for women. There was no significant difference by age either.

There is a stark contrast between this community and the general population regarding weight. According to the National Institute of Health, 30.7% of adults are overweight, or about 1 in 3 adults. About 2 in 5 adults (42.4%) have obesity. Combine 42.4 % with the 9.1 % of young people under age the age of 20 who are obese brings the total to 51.5 %. In other words, half of the population is obese (that is, people with a body mass index of 25 or above). Obesity is defined as having a BMI greater than or equal to 30. Whereas, in this Amish community, there were only 4 % who would be considered obese.15 (If you want to calculate your BMI, divide your weight by the number of inches in height. Take the result of that calculation and divide it by your height in inches again. Then, multiply that result by 703 to get the BMI. For example, Weight = 150 lbs., Height = 5'5" (65 inches) BMI Calculation: [150 ÷ (65)2] x 703 = 24.96)

So, God's wisdom about the benefits of work is multifaceted. It is not just about financial benefits; it is also about physical benefits. Remember the statement that these wisdom teachings *"are life to those who find them. They are health to your whole body"* (Proverbs 4:22 NIrV). With all of this in mind, when we read the following passages about work, we gain greater insight into how beneficial work is for one's well-being.

"From the fruit of their lips people are filled with good things, and the work of their hands brings them reward" (Proverbs 12:14). *"All hard work brings a profit, but mere talk leads only to poverty"* (Proverbs 14:23). *"I went past the field of a sluggard, past the vineyard of someone who has no sense; thorns had come up everywhere, the ground was covered with weeds, and the stone wall was in ruins. I applied my heart to what I observed and learned a lesson from what I saw: A little sleep, a little slumber, a little folding of the hands to rest—and poverty will come on you like a thief and scarcity like an armed man"* (Proverbs 24:30–34).

The Centers for Disease Control and Prevention recommend 150 minutes of moderate activity each week or 30 minutes of walking each day, as well as two days of muscle-strengthening activity.[108] How many steps would you take if you walked the recommended 30-minute daily walk? Neil Johannsen, assistant Professor in the School of Kinesiology at Louisiana State University, says some research indicates about 7,500 steps per day would be the total with a 30-minute walk included each day.

Sedentary people in the U.S. generally move only two to three thousand steps daily. Older adults and those with chronic diseases typically take 3,500 to 5,500 steps daily. In one study, healthy older adults, who were sixty-nine years old and older, took about 6,600 steps per day, with almost 3,000 steps coming from structured, planned movement or about one-and-a-half miles per day.[109]

Research indicates that 10,000 steps or more per day is beneficial to health. One study with hypertensive patients found that walking 10,000 steps daily lowered their blood pressure, increased exercise capacity, and reduced sympathetic nerve activity. The sympathetic nervous system accelerates the heart rate, constricts blood vessels, and raises blood pressure. This was not dependent on the intensity of the exercise or duration.[110] Another four-week 10,000-step study of overweight women showed improvement in blood glucose control and blood pressure even with no changes in body mass, body fat percentage, or waist circumference.[111]

In Dr. Casey Means book "Good Energy: The Surprising Connection Between Metabolism and Limitless Heath" she writes this about the significance of walking 10,000 steps per day. *"Simply walking about 10,000 steps per day (as compared with lower amounts) is associated with the following:*

- 50 percent lower dementia risk
- 50 to 70 percent lower risk of premature death
- 44 percent lower risk of getting type 2 diabetes
- 31 percent (or more) lower risk of obesity
- 50 percent lower dementia risk

- significant reductions in cancer occurrence, major depression, gastric reflux, and sleep apnea.

Zero medications or surgeries can do for chronic disease prevention what walking about 10,000 steps a day can do. Despite this, physicians rarely prescribe exercise to patients. If a medication could slash Alzheimer's risk by 50 percent, it would be front-page news and prescribed to every patient. But this "drug" does exist—it's walking!" [112]

So, would taking more steps each day be worth it? Of course, it would! First, find out your average number of steps per day using a pedometer or a fitness tracker like a Fitbit. After wearing a pedometer for a few days and finding your average number of steps daily, set your initial goal—6600, 7500, or 10000 or more steps per day. Put on your pedometer first thing in the morning and take it off right before going to bed, or just wear a fitness tracker all day and night (these devices also monitor the quality and amount of sleep—more about sleep in chapter 7). Start adding a few steps each day until you reach your goal. Adding a few steps each day is the best approach. The way of wisdom teaches the power of the little by a little method. *"Money that comes easily disappears quickly, but money that is gathered little by little will grow"* (Proverbs 13:11 NCV). Remember, *"For the LORD gives wisdom; from his mouth come knowledge and understanding. He holds success in store for the upright"* (Proverbs 2:6-7).

Mitochondria

Someone says, "I'm always tired. I have no energy!" *"Plans fail for lack of counsel, but with many advisers they succeed"* (Proverbs

15:22). *"For lack of guidance a nation falls, but victory is won through many advisers"* (Proverbs 11:14). If you read and put into practice the following advice, you will be practicing God's wisdom with rich results for more energy!

How long can you breathe before becoming fatigued? Have you ever thought about that? As you read this, you are still breathing. You aren't exhausted, and that is because of the abundance of mitochondria in the muscle cells. They are tiny energy producers. Dr. Mark Hyman says this. "Mitochondria are key energy sources for our bodies. They are tiny factories housed within our cells that take the foods we eat and the oxygen we breathe and convert them into energy. That energy is called adenosine triphosphate, or ATP, and it is used to support every function in our bodies. Each cell holds hundreds or thousands of mitochondria; they are found in greater concentrations in active organs and tissues like the heart, brain, and muscles. In fact, we have more than 100,000 trillion mitochondria in our bodies, and each one contains 17,000 little assembly lines for making ATP. Mitochondria are where metabolism happens."[113] ATP stands for adenosine triphosphate. It is the energy source. When we break down the word triphosphate, the tri is three phosphate molecules. They are bound together, and energy is released when the mitochondria break them apart.

Cellular respiration is the process by which mitochondria combine food with oxygen to form ATP. The mitochondria are like factories with assembly lines. Nutrients assist the production line of food and oxygen. They are like workers and tools for the product—the energy.[114]

When we think of this, we see how relevant the psalmist's

words are. *"I praise you because you made me in an amazing and wonderful way. What you have done is wonderful. I know this very well"* (Psalm 139:14).

Your breathing muscles' activity is aerobic because the mitochondria aid the cells as tiny energy producers, providing oxygen and fatigue resistance. So, when we start walking, the leg muscles do not fatigue because they are abundant with mitochondria. When you walk, there is a response for less insulin needed, which can last for up to 48 hours. Insulin resistance reverses, and blood sugar comes down.[115]

When I walk, I speed up my pace and even jog for half a block. This is called **interval training** or intermittently speeding up the pace. People with Type 2 Diabetes who usually walked 10,000 steps daily participated in a twelve-week study of picking up the pace for part of their daily steps. They walked their typical 10,000 steps but increased their speed for part of their walks. As a result, they experienced an increase in how well their insulin worked—insulin sensitivity. Dr. Colberg, an exercise expert with Type 1 Diabetes, mentions several good benefits of this exercise, such as burning more fat and glucose, improving blood glucose control, strengthening the heart, and extending the calorie-burning power of muscles after workouts.[116]

When we pick up the pace another benefit is to strengthen the energy structures in the cell, the mitochondria. The older we get, the less effective the cells' mitochondria become in producing energy. Research on seventy-two people without diabetes, thirty-six from ages 18 to 30 and thirty-six from 65 to 80, discovered that through high-intensity interval biking, mitochondria capacity increases. The high-intensity Interval training saw a 49% increase in mitochondrial capacity, and the older volunteers saw an even more dramatic 69% increase.[117] What does this do? An increase in capacity results in more energy and helps us live a longer, healthier life.

People with Type 2 Diabetes have difficulties with weight control, elevated blood glucose (sugar), dysfunctional mitochondria, fatigue and insulin resistance. Insulin resistance is a key component of type 2 diabetes. Several research studies link the dysfunction of mitochondria in skeletal muscle to the development of insulin resistance.[118] Research on people with Type 2 Diabetes between the ages of 30 and 55 who lead sedentary lifestyles indicated that through weight loss and weekly exercise, all of these dysfunctions can be reversed. In this research, the participants performed moderate weekly exercise consistent with a healthy lifestyle. The study lasted about twenty weeks. Most participants chose walking on a treadmill as their exercise. They began with thirty minutes for the first month and then increased to forty minutes for the second month.

A 7% mean reduction in weight, with nearly all subjects losing at least 5% of their weight, resulted in better insulin sensitivity. Besides the weight loss, an even better predictor for insulin sensitivity was the energy expended in exercise sessions. Their research demonstrated that lifestyle changes can improve the muscle mitochondria.[119] More research indicates that the following changes will also improve mitochondria's capacity to function and give the most energy. Besides exercise, let's consider five more ways to do this, like calorie restriction (fasting), nutrients like vitamin B (Spinach, kale, Brussels sprouts, cabbage, broccoli, and turnip greens), Omega 3 fats (salmon, chia seeds, flax seeds, walnuts, and egg yolks), sleep, and sunlight (vitamin D).

Some studies show that during fasting and intermittent fasting, the body repairs damaged mitochondria and even makes more, improving mitochondrial health. Research trials of overweight women who used intermittent fasting two days per week resulted in more significant increases in insulin sensitivity, and greater losses of weight in the waistline than those who cut calories by twenty-five percent.[120] Both lost the same weight, but waistline fat causes greater insulin resistance. Also significant at the cellular level, fasting increases antioxidant defenses and mitochondrial biogenesis, which are more of them.[121]

Here is how to practice intermittent fasting. After trying Time-Restricted Eating in the evenings, you could restrict eating all morning. In other words, fast until noon or one. Then, you would have a window to eat for the next six hours. I've done this successfully for better blood sugar control and weight loss. There are several things to consider when trying an 18:6 or 16:8 (fasting for 16 to 18 hours and having an eating window from six to eight hours) fasting schedule. Sixteen hours may seem long, but if you're getting adequate sleep, you should be asleep for about seven hours.

Another thing we need to do during those morning hours is not succumb to temptations. Keep snack food out of reach and out of sight. By doing this, you can persevere and reap great rewards for your health. *"Let us not become weary in doing good, for at the proper time we will reap a harvest if we do not give up"*

(Galatians 6: 9). What is happening with your body as you fast? It helps to know so that you can endure and not give up. Here is a basic outline of what I've read happens. For the first eight hours, blood sugars fall, food has left the stomach, and the body produces minimal insulin for basal metabolisms like breathing and the heart. Does your BMR stop working during sickness? "The basal metabolic rate, or BMR, is the amount of energy required to support the work of the heart, brain, lungs, and other organs at rest without any physical or mental exertion," says Boris Draznin, M.D. Then, the digestive system sleeps for the next four hours, the body begins healing, and human growth hormone increases. This what happens for hours fourteen through eighteen.

Food consumed has been burned, the digestive system goes to sleep, the body begins the healing process, human growth hormone increases, and glucagon is relaxed to balance blood sugars during the twelve and thirteen hours. After fourteen hours, the body has converted to using stored fat as energy and human growth hormone increases dramatically.[122]

Then God said, "I give you every seed-bearing plant on the face of the whole earth and every tree that has fruit with seed in it. They will be yours for food. And to all the beasts of the earth and all the birds in the sky and all the creatures that move along the ground—everything that has the breath of life in it—I give every green plant for food." And it was so (Genesis 1:29-30).

Nutrients like vitamin B (Spinach, kale, Brussels sprouts, cabbage, broccoli, and turnip greens) can help keep your mitochondria healthy. The mitochondria are like factories with assembly lines. The production line with food and oxygen is assisted by nutrients, the workers, and the tools for the prod-uct—the energy.

Eat whole foods and avoid processed foods with empty calo-ries. Think of an assembly line with tools and workers. Nutrients like B vitamins, vitamin C, zinc, and chromium are some of the essential workers on the production line of our mitochondria. They are like the nutrients that generate energy. When they brake down or are absent, they impact ATP production.[123]

When we sleep we are not just dreaming and wasting time. Our bodies are designed to use that time to stay or get healthy! Several processes are happening as we sleep. According to the National Sleep Foundation, such health ben-efits as "muscle repair, memory consolidation and release of hormones regulating growth and appetite" are happening. This prepares us to concentrate and **make decisions for all day time activities.** As we sleep, we go through several stages of sleep. These stages repeat throughout the night in about ninety-minute cycles. Our bodies are as the psalmist writes, *"Fearfully and wonderfully made"* (Psalm 139: 14). **Physical health is also impacted by sleep deprivation.** There is an impairment of hormones that relate to appetite. Less leptin, the "feel full" hormone is released, and more of ghrelin, the "still hungry" hormone. This makes losing weight an even greater challenge. So, the strategy is to sleep more and lose weight.[124] Studies also reveal that cortisol levels increase the next evening after just one night of sleep loss, causing insu-lin resistance. Also, the efficiency of the immune response is damaged as well as an increase in inflammation with lack of sleep.[125] A lack of sleep also lowers the levels of the chemical serotonin, which then results in pain sensitivity increasing as well as increased feelings of anxiety. To compensate for lower levels, the body compensates with cravings for carbohydrates.[126] Another factor of sleep deprivation is cell stress or oxidative stress. Scientific Research indicates that free radicals escape from your mitochondria and attack your cells. Free radicals are produced while you're awake and are eliminated when you sleep. Sleep deprivation inhibits your body's ability to fight cell stress.[127]

So how can we get a good night's sleep. God's wisdom says this. *"My son, do not let wisdom and understanding out of your sight... When you lie down, you will not be afraid; when you lie down, your sleep will be sweet... When you walk, they will guide you; when you sleep, they will watch over you; when you awake, they will speak to you."* (Proverbs 3: 21, 24; 6: 22).

"Whoever seeks good finds favor, but evil comes to one who searches for it" (Proverbs 11: 27). By seeking what is good, listing the good, meditating on the good are all practices of keeping wisdom in sight. These are all methods for having sweet sleep. What can easily happen instead of focusing on the good is to focus on problems or worries. Thinking about them over and over again is not conducive to falling asleep. In fact, by meditating on them they are compounded and become independent of reality. These worries can easily become worse and more powerful than they are. This all leads to restlessness, not seeing live clearly, and mounting obstacles and hazards for falling asleep. Dwelling on what is good will fight off the anxiety of worry. *"A cheerful look brings joy to your heart. And good news gives health to your body"* (Proverbs 15: 30 NIrV).

One more factor to consider for mitochondria health is **sunlight.** It provides Vitamin D plus D sulphate which only the sun can provide. Ten to twenty minutes of sunlight is what is needed to for mitochondrial function.[128] **Omega 3 fats** (salmon, chia seeds, flax seeds, walnuts, and egg yolks) are also helpful in keeping mitochondria healthy and functional.

Mayo Clinic Research Study

Dr. James Levine of the Mayo Clinic conducted an extensive eight-week study in which sixteen people with sedentary lifestyles were fed exactly a thousand extra calories per day. Each participant ate an extra 56,000 calories, which equals a weight gain of sixteen pounds. What were the results?

One person barely gained an ounce. By contrast, one lady gained fourteen pounds! Everyone else was in between those extremes. How could some people barely gain any weight? Where were all those extra calories going? They had to be shedding all those calories daily, but how? They were not allowed to start a walking program, either. No one went out and walked several miles each night.

Ethan was the guy who didn't gain any weight. How did he do it? Was he sneaking in exercise or doing a midnight marathon? No! He didn't even realize it, but he had started moving more. Instead of driving his son to the bus stop, he walked him. He started pacing up and down the sidelines during his son's soccer games. He even got up in the middle of the night and did little things, like adjust the drapes or shut the window. He didn't even remember those actions, but his wife did and told him about them. In this Mayo Clinic overfeeding study, those who didn't gain weight responded by spontaneously moving more.[11]

Why does spontaneously moving help? Dr. Levine at the Mayo Clinic informs us that our capillaries are lined with special cells (endothelial), which contain an enzyme (lipoprotein lipase LPL) that breaks down fat molecules (triglycerides) in the blood. These enzymes start to switch off when we sit for a few hours. The mere act of getting up out of a chair breaks them out of hibernation mode.[12]

Watch: Dr. Levine explain his research at "James Levine, M.D., Ph.D.—Transform 2010—Mayo Clinic **https://www. youtube.com/watch?v=S6elvxqaezE**

More Moving Suggestions

Instead of parking your car as close to the front entrance of a store as you can, why not park your vehicle way back in the corner of the parking lot, where the people with brand-new cars park theirs? It allows you to put more steps on your pedometer. A small activity, like standing up and stretching during the commercials of a basketball or football game you're watching, can make a difference. Mowing the lawn, sweeping the sidewalk, raking leaves, walking up and down a flight of stairs, or just standing more will help burn more calories. The following four examples show the benefits of moving more.

"I went past the field of a sluggard, past the vineyard of someone who has no sense; thorns had come up everywhere, the ground was covered with weeds, and the stone wall was in ruins. I applied my heart to what I observed and learned a lesson from what I saw: A little sleep, a little slumber, a little folding of the hands to rest—and

poverty will come on you like a thief and scarcity like an armed man" (Proverbs 24:30–34).

Hard Work

What does God's wisdom say about work? *"Those who work their land will have abundant food, but those who chase fantasies have no sense...From the fruit of their lips people are filled with good things, and the work of their hands brings them reward... All hard work brings a profit, but mere talk leads only to poverty"* (Proverbs 12:11,14, 14:23). Work brings monetary and material rewards, but the common work in 1000 BC, the time these proverbs were written, brought another type of reward. Here is an example of that type of work. *"Let me go to the fields and pick up the leftover grain behind anyone in whose eyes I find favor." Naomi said to her, "Go ahead, my daughter." So she went out, entered a field and began to glean behind the harvesters. As it turned out, she was working in a field belonging to Boaz* (Ruth 2:2-3). This type of work would bring monetary rewards, but this type of work would also bring another type of reward— physical health. Moving, lifting, turning, guiding a plow with an ox, and harvesting a crop by hand would all be common activities then. Images like that would come to people's minds as they thought of these proverbs. Sitting in front of a desk would not enter the mind of the wise, but rather standing and moving jobs would—manual labor!

When thinking about the benefits of work, the following news headline grabbed my attention: "A father and his sons cut wood to fill 80 trucks. Then they brought it to homes that needed heat."[129] That headline was meaningful because these men were not doing this to benefit themselves but rather to help the needy.

At first, this forty-seven-year-old father and his twenty-one-year-old twin sons were chopping together as a family activity. They like to chop wood; it is a family tradition. The father did it with his father and he has passed the tradition on to his sons. Last summer they started chopping and the wood kept accumulating until it reached a value of over 15,000 dollars. In Washington State where they live, 20-degree temperatures were coming in early November. They could easily start selling wood, but instead, they decided to post it as "free" on Facebook and see what would happen. They got request after request from people in real need. They not only gave it away but also during the evenings they would even deliver the wood.

They began bringing wood to hundreds of needy people who do not have money to buy it. They began helping some of the neediest people in their area, who only use wood to heat their homes. One single mom, living in a mobile home with only a wood-burning stove for heat, was overwhelmed with the generosity. She said, "To get that much wood and the chimney sweep brought me to tears. So much stress and anxiety for my daughter is off my shoulders. I couldn't be more thankful."

These three men are often met with tears and hugs of heartfelt gratitude as they make deliveries. The father, Shane McDaniel, said something very insightful, "It has nothing to do with how well it's received, but it's about how much it's needed."

This is an impressive story of hard work and generosity. It reminds me of what Luke wrote about Paul. *"In everything I did, I showed you that by this kind of hard work we must help the weak, remembering the words the Lord Jesus himself said: 'It is more blessed to give than to receive'"* (Acts 20:35).

> *It is a sin to despise one's neighbor, but blessed is the*
> *one who is kind to the needy* (Proverbs 14:21).

107 Years and Working Hard

One person allows only one barber to cut his hair because of his experience. He says, "This guy's been cutting hair for a century." That was an exaggeration because he's only been cutting hair for ninety-six years. Mr. Mancinelli started in 1921 when Warren G. Harding was president. He has cut hair for generations—fathers, grandfathers, great-grandfathers. Some customers have been coming to him for more than fifty years, getting hundreds of haircuts from just him.[130]

Yes, he has experience starting in 1921 as a boy of about 11 and continuing to this day at 107 years old. Longevity is what usually happens when people use a wise "common sense" approach to life. *"Blessed are those who find wisdom... Long life is in her right hand"* (Proverbs 3:13, 16).

His very example is an inspiration to some of his older customers. His son relates his favorite phrase for eighty-year-old customers is "Listen, when you get to be my age..." That's encouragement, and "they love hearing it." *"Worry weighs a person down; an encouraging word cheers a person up... A cheerful heart is good medicine, but a crushed spirit dries up the bones"* (Proverbs 12:25, 17:22).

He works hard, never calls in sick and even sweeps up the hair clippings himself. He continues to work and keeps busy five days a week from noon until 8 p.m. He works Saturdays when it is most busy. A young fellow worker said she gets tired being on her feet all day "but he just keeps going." *"All hard work brings a profit, but mere talk leads only to poverty"* (Proverbs 14:23).

To stay busy and work full-time helps him to stay upbeat after the loss of his wife fourteen years ago. He misses her and goes to her grave every day before going to work. Loyal is what he is to his work and as well as to his wife of sixty-nine years. *"Many claim to have unfailing love, but a faithful person who can find?"* (Proverbs 20:6).

Many people ask about his secret to longevity and his simple answer is to just put in a satisfying day of work. He also uses a wise "common sense" approach to what he eats, avoiding harmful drinks and foods. He claims he stays thin by eating thin spaghetti. From the way of wisdom, the "common sense" approach to life includes the following: *"From the fruit of their lips people are filled with good things, and the work of their hands brings them reward... Lazy people want much but get little, but those who work hard will prosper... The wisdom of the prudent is to give thought to their ways"* (Proverbs 12:14, 13:4, 14:8). Sounds like a good approach for wise living! Patient, too, with the variety of clients he's had in almost a century. He died on Sept 19, 2019, at his home in New Windsor, N.Y., a Hudson River town about an hour's drive north of New York City. He was 108. His son, Bob, 82, said the cause was jaw cancer. His father had retired, reluctantly, only weeks before. "He didn't know the meaning of the word retired," Bob Mancinelli said. That is being on his feet and being very patient in his work.

Watch: "This 107-Year-Old Is the World's Oldest Barber" at https://www.youtube.com/watch?v=B9jH-3ylTAk

Movement Motivation: A Walk to the Hospital

Some people can do amazing things. Walking six miles round trip from home to the hospital would not be surprising for a man in his twenties. To be ninety-nine and walk that distance each day is quite remarkable.

Most people would accept a ride if offered or take the bus. Luther does neither. He's done a lot of walking in his life since his work involved manual labor. He also says the walk clears his mind. Those are not the real motivating factors for his determination to walk to the hospital each day. What motivates him is his love for his wife. They've been married for fifty-five years now, and he doesn't want her to be there by herself. His wife was diagnosed with a brain tumor in 2009. She has been in and out of the hospital; her most current stay has been for three months. Her bedside is where he belongs, and so he walks. On one occasion, a reporter walked with him. As he got closer to the hospital, he even picked up his pace and began to run.[131]

The love for his wife gives him the willpower to walk no matter the weather. His walking is not just because he loves her but also because she loves him. He says, "She's my wife; she's my best friend." When he says walking clears his mind, what remains in his mind is his wife's love for him. Their daughter says, "He's always cared about her the way he does [now]. He loves my mom. He'll do anything for her." This story is not about walking for exercise, although walking is important for health. Luther says he doesn't smoke, doesn't drink. He attributes that to his health also. The love he and his wife have for each other is what makes the difference.

Love is a great motivator. With love, amazing things can happen. The apostle John referred to himself as *"the disciple whom Jesus loved"* (John 21:20). He writes in his first letter *"Dear friends, let us love one another, for love comes from God... Whoever does not love does not know God, because God is love... This is love: not that we loved God, but that he loved us and sent his Son as an atoning sacrifice for our sins. Dear friends, since God so loved us, we also ought to love one another"* (1 John 4:7-8, 10-11). And Solomon writes, *"My son, do not forget my teaching, but keep my commands in your heart, for they will prolong your life many years and bring you peace and prosperity. Let love and faithfulness never leave you; bind them around your neck, write them on the tablet of your heart. Then you will win favor and a good name in the sight of God and man"* (Proverbs 3:1-4).

Watch: 99-Year-Old Walks 6 Miles a Day to Visit His Wife in the Hospital **https://www.youtube.com/watch?v=Tb_-PHZO4rE**

CHAPTER NINE

Encourage Others

Additional information on # 17—
Take advantage of opportunities to help others.

Rescue, observe, care, safety, and frantic are all words that fit an alarming event in the news. A deputy saw an unbelievable sight while traveling at night on an Oregon highway. He thought it was some animal running down the middle of the road. His dashboard camera was recording it all as he got closer. He was stunned to see a two-year-old boy running down the highway. The toddler was in danger. The deputy slammed on his brakes. He immediately got out of his car and scooped up the boy as a semi-truck passed nearby.

A tragic story could have unfolded if the deputy had been distracted and not carefully observing the road that night. That little boy, however, was rescued and brought to safety. The deputy's swift and observant actions averted a potential disaster. The deputy soon discovered that his parents were frantically looking for him. He had slipped out of a nearby community center while his parents were cleaning.

Watch: "Toddler found running down busy highway is saved by police officer" at **https://www.youtube.com/watch?v=sni8_4BhqRk**

That little boy is like so many people running down the highway of life. They need help! What would you do if you saw a toddler walking on the road? Without hesitation, you would stop and rescue him! The Lord tells us, *"What is desirable in a man is his kindness"* (Proverbs 19:22 NASB). We all want kindness from others. Kindness is appreciated. Kindness toward a lost toddler should be easy. Transferring that attitude toward others is needed.

A gem found in God's wisdom is this: *"A **generous** person will **prosper**; whoever refreshes others will be refreshed"* (Proverbs 11:25). The Hebrew word translated as "prosper" means "to be fat, grow fat, become fat, become prosperous." In other words, in contrast to skin and bones, "prosper" is healthy, not wealthy!

We've all found times when we need refreshment in life! Have you ever been in a hospital bed, asking for help, and no one comes? When ignored, anguish can result. I've been there! I read about a surgeon who became the patient. The doctor was recovering from surgery, immobile, and needed a helping hand. Surprisingly, he received it at the start of the 6:30 morning shift. In walks, a nurse making her morning rounds, checking on him. She is about to leave, but then she suddenly stops! She goes over to the sink and moistens a clean washcloth with warm water. She then goes to him and wipes his face. All she says is, "This must be hard for you." In this lonely hospital room, someone paused to reflect on his feelings, to sympathize with his burden with these precious, sparse words, "This must be hard for you." Those six words made a difference for him! She was generous, refreshing him with just six words, showing that kindness can be as simple as a few words and a warm washcloth.

> *"A good person gives life to others; the wise person teaches others how to live"* (Proverbs 11:30 NCV).

To Be Encouraged, Encourage

When I was recovering from back surgery, a laminectomy in 1988, I was kept in a wing of a large hospital just for patients with diabetes. I was thirty-five. During my stay of ten days, I discovered five people with Type 1 Diabetes who were already blind from the complication of retinopathy; four were younger than me and one about five years older. It took me almost thirty years to realize how serious this disease is. I saw it. Two years before this I had a massive hemorrhage in my right eye. So, I resolved to help people, to help them feel better every day, to support them so that they wouldn't have to face such devastating complications. That decision helped me get better control of my diabetes as well.

In the fall of 1992, I started a diabetes support group at the Good Samaritan Hospital in Kearney, Nebraska. For the first meeting, thirty-five attended. I introduced myself, and for the next several years, I gave encouraging support to those who attended, helping hundreds of people. For the last thirty years, I've continued to facilitate either hospital or community diabetes support groups where ever I've lived.

Many people will not admit they have diabetes or any chronic disease. Their disease is private, their secret. What is missed with that attitude? What is missed is their opportunity to not only help others but to help themselves! Eventually the hospital in Kearney, Nebraska hired a Certified Diabetes Educator. One day, I received a call from her, telling me there was a noncompliant patient with Type 1 diabetes in the hospital. Would I visit him? I agreed. He would not cooperate, even putting the sheets over his head when they entered his room. When I asked to enter his room, identifying myself as a fellow Type 1, he invited me in and opened up to me.

We talked about the challenges we were both facing. He was finding great difficulty in keeping his blood sugar under control. He had never had any support or encouragement. His mom was not helpful. Friends of hers had even influenced him to drink. So, after he was released from the hospital, he attended the support group meetings. We also met weekly. I shared portions from a book called "Diabetes: A Guide to Living Well" by Dr. Gary Arsham. Dr. Arsham was diagnosed with Type 1 diabetes when he was ten. Unlike today, there were few books available for people with diabetes in 1994. So, in a sense, he became part of our weekly meetings. People need encouragement. Randy started doing better with his blood sugar levels, but he already had kidney failure. He started on Peritoneal Dialysis.

Not only did we use the diabetes guide book, but we looked at encouraging Proverbs like *"The fear of the LORD is the beginning of wisdom, and knowledge of the Holy One is understanding. For through wisdom your days will be many, and years will be added to your life. If you are wise, your wisdom will reward you"* (Proverbs

9:10-12). He started coming to Bible class. When he started his mom wanted to know why in the world he was doing that. He said because he had never tried it before. He was trying a lot of new things like routinely checking his blood sugar. He wanted to see if attending Bible class would make a difference. And it did!

One day after eating lunch together, as we traveled toward my office, we saw a lawn that really needed mowing. The person who lived there was a widow, a recluse whose husband had died in World War 2. I casually said we should just go mow her lawn. After saying that, I went on a trip out of state. When I got back, I discovered Randy had taken his mower in the trunk of his car and mowed the whole lawn, taking the cuttings to the dump yard. I asked if she ever said anything to him. She only said, "What are you doing?" No, thanks, no gratitude! Randy was practicing God's wisdom. *"Blessed is the one who is kind to the needy"* (Proverbs 14:21). That is the kind of behavior a Christian should have. So, a few days later he became a Christian, being baptized into Christ (read Acts 22:16, Galatians 3:27, Romans 6:3-4).

Randy was on a kidney transplant list, and not long after, this wonderful news arrived—a kidney and pancreas. When he received that pancreas, he was no longer in the community of diabetics. This good news was countered with bad news because within a few weeks, he was in a car/train wreck. The train won. He was flown to Omaha with a broken femur, ribs, and arm and severe trauma to his head. He was in rehab for months. How did he stay encouraged during those weeks of therapy? He focused on good things. He said just as Paul walked on water, as long as he kept his eyes on Jesus (it was actually Peter), he was encouraged and strengthened. Here is a question he asked me. What is the most rewarding thing about your job? "What is most rewarding," I said, "is when I see people encouraged and helped!"

Look for people you can encourage. For example, start a walking club! One woman at our diabetes support group knew she needed to start walking. She needed motivation! She asked at a support group meeting if anyone would meet her at the park to help her get started. Three people volunteered. But instead of just three showing up, twelve did! Can you imagine how it would be to show up to walk and have about a dozen others there to help you get started? It would be encouraging and motivating! I've discovered that when I look for people I can encourage and support, they've helped me, too! Those who showed up to help her get started walking walked, too. So, in a sense, she was helping them, also. When we look for others to support, we, too, will be encouraged! Being blessed and refreshed will result just as Jesus and Solomon said: *"It is more blessed to give than to receive...A generous person will prosper; whoever refreshes others will be refreshed"* (Acts 20:35, Proverbs 11:25).

Albert: Obscure Significance

Many noteworthy people work for the health of people at hospitals, like physicians, surgeons, nurses, and a polisher of shoes—polisher of shoes? Yes, a polisher of shoes was significant. He worked at a hospital shining shoes for twenty-eight years, making about ten thousand dollars a year. He worked at the Children's Hospital of Pittsburgh starting in 1981 and retiring in 2013. During those twenty-eight years, he received over 202,000 dollars in tips but didn't keep a penny for himself. Instead, he donated every dollar to the "Free Care Fund." That fund ensures that children who need medical care receive it whether their families can pay or not.

This man, Albert Lexie, passed away recently at the age of 76. He would get up at 5:50 every morning and would be at work by 7:25 each day for twenty-eight years. His purpose was not just to shine shoes but rather to donate every tip he received to benefit sick, uninsured children. The hospital's president said about Lexie that he was "a perfect example of how just small, incremental acts of kindness can have a significant impact over time."[132] Let's keep doing the small obscure acts of kindness too because they can make a difference in the lives of people! *"Always try to be kind to each other and to everyone else"* (1 Thessalonians 5:15).

> **Watch:** "Pittsburgh Shoe shiner donates $200K in tips to Needy Children" **https://www.youtube.com/watch?v=D4nFAjJy2f8**

Unusual Resolutions

"Everyone has a future; some plan theirs." Some people make resolutions, but few keep them. Some research indicates that about 62% of people make New Year's resolutions, but only 8% achieve them. If people could achieve their resolutions, they would be very beneficial and meaningful like in spending less and saving more, staying fit and healthy, helping others and spending more time with family.

None of the examples mentioned are unusual. However,

have you ever heard of a person making a New Year's Resolution to donate a kidney to an unknown person in need? That is not a normal resolution! When the need was noticed, she kept her resolution too.

David's kidneys had shut down; he was on kidney dialysis. The dialysis had started five years ago when he was only twenty-four. He wasn't handling his situation very well. He knew he was not in a good frame of mind and that his situation was tough, and getting tougher. He was on a donor's list, which doctors said could take years to find a match. Proverbs 18:14 was coming true in him. *"A man's spirit sustains him in sickness, but a crushed spirit who can bear?"*

He decided to try one more place, so he asked for help on Craigslist. Asking is the principle Jesus teaches on the "sermon on the mount" when he said, *"Ask and it will be given to you; seek and you will find; knock and the door will be opened to you. For everyone who asks receives; the one who seeks finds; and to the one who knocks, the door will be opened"* (Matthew 7:7-8). When David put an ad on Craigslist asking for a kidney, he got several responses. Most were foreign donors wanting money and help in immigrating to America, but one stood out.[133]

Jessica, the twenty-nine-year-old surgical nurse, responded. She was the one who had made the resolution she intended to keep. David, at first, thought her response was just another scam. Testing proved they were a match. On June 14, his situation improved as he received a kidney that changed his life. He does not look at Jessica as a fraud, but rather, he sees her as a "gift from God." Let's remember, we are to *"walk in the way of love"* (Ephesians 5:2). We are to *"always try to be kind to each other and to everyone else"* (1 Thessalonians 5:15). Kindness comes in many plans, as shown through Jessica.

Longevity

Willard Scott, as weatherman on the Today show, was best known for his weather forecasts and for greeting those turning one hundred years old throughout the United States. He started this practice way back in 1983. Celebrating the age of 100 grabbed peoples' attention back then, and it still does.

A longtime Chick-fil-A customer, Steve, turned 100 in 2018. He would come to this restaurant for breakfast every day for twenty years. He would order the same food, sit at the same booth, read his paper, and visit with employees each morning. His presence was a daily highlight for them. This Chick-fil-A honored his 100th birthday with a CFA for life. In addition, they had a special celebration for his 100th birthday, which garnered national attention, allowing him to star in a commercial filmed in New York City.

It is always interesting to hear what others think of individuals who turn a hundred years old. Some Facebook posts read, "His visit was a daily highlight and our team would carve out a good five to ten minutes each day to sit and talk with him." He is the "sweetest, most genuine, kind, and humble person we have had the pleasure to know." They just celebrated his 104th birthday, and this is what they wrote. "As we celebrated 104, we couldn't help but feel immensely grateful for the opportunity to return even a portion of the love that he shares with our team, and for the bond that we have been able to build over the past six years of birthdays."

Chick-fil-A employees expressed kindness and humility as two characteristics of 104-year-old Steve. What does God's wisdom say about longevity? *"For through wisdom your days will be many, and years will be added to your life. If you are wise, your wisdom will reward you"* (Proverbs 9:11-12). We shouldn't be surprised that kindness and humility are the teachings of God's wisdom. *"Your own soul is nourished when you are kind"* (Proverbs 11:17).

Yes, God's wisdom works for longevity. *"Long life is in her right hand; in her left hand are riches and honor. Her ways are pleasant ways, and all her paths are peace. She is a tree of life to those who take hold of her; those who hold her fast will be blessed"* (Proverbs 3:16-18). *"Go to the ant, you sluggard; consider its ways and be wise! It has no commander, no overseer or ruler, yet it stores its provisions in summer and gathers its food at harvest"* (Proverbs 6:16-18). Let's use that wisdom as motivation to live a long life.

Goodness in a 100-Year-Old

The day a woman turns 100, she is honored to throw the ceremonial pitch at a professional baseball game. She says she has waited 100 years to throw the pitch. "I never could have imagined celebrating a birthday like this, let alone my 100th," says Helen Kahan of St. Petersburg, Florida. We can understand how amazing this is once we realize she survived three Nazi concentration camps and escaped from a death march in Nazi-occupied Germany.

With a great depth of understanding and insight, she says the following: "I'm so grateful that I am here to tell my story and help the world remember why kindness and empathy are so important for us all." In the Holocaust, she lost her parents, sisters, brothers, and grandmothers." After experiencing such horrible circumstances, becoming bitter, resentful, and filled with hate would be easy. The 100-year-old Helen chose a different path, a path the proverb describes in this way. *"The path of the righteous is like the morning sun, shining ever brighter till the full light of day"* (Proverbs 4:18).

The Holocaust showed the worst of evil, but some people like Helen found a way to stay positive despite it. People describe her as a "sunny person." She lives her life with appreciation, being grateful for surviving even though so many others, including her family, didn't. She remembers growing up in a happy family. This is her advice for living a good life. "Be strong and help everybody." "Be **good** to people and just do the best you can do." Helen has been doing good since those terrible days of World War II. She married another Holocaust survivor, and they raised two daughters. Her family has expanded with five grandchildren and twelve great-grandchildren.[134]

Her words remind me of Paul's instructions. He encourages Titus, *"In everything set them an example by doing what is **good**"* (Titus 2:7). Paul also writes this. *"Our people must learn to devote themselves to doing what is **good**, in order to provide for urgent needs and not live unproductive lives"* (Titus 3:14). The Greek Lexicon on the word *good*—καλός kalos means "right or beautiful." People can do ugly, disgusting, hideous acts that are so cruel, but we need to see what is beautiful. Paul gives this instruction on how to overcome such things. *"Do not be overcome by evil, but overcome evil with good"* (Romans 12:21). Before that statement, he gives an example from the Proverbs. *"If your enemy is hungry,* *feed him; if he is thirsty, give him something to drink. In doing this, you will heap burning coals on his head."* Let's practice goodness and overcome evil!

Traveling and Helping

Traveling the road toward Boise, Idaho, a gust of wind caused the driver to over-compensate, lose control of the car and flip it off the road. The driver of a van behind that car saw all of this happen. At first, he only saw kicked-up dust, not knowing the car's condition. As the dust settled, he stopped and noticed the overturned car. He told the six others in the van to stay put until he could go and see the extent of the tragedy. He hoped he wouldn't see anything gruesome, and as he didn't, he called six youth football offensive linemen out of the van. They were thirteen or fourteen years old. To rescue the passenger, Alan Hardeman, they partially lifted the car. He had passed out in the crash, but "young voices" were trying to help wake him.[135]

His wife was still stuck behind the steering wheel. A second van soon arrived, loaded with more football players. This team had just won a California championship tournament. Their season was 11-0, but this rescue event gave these players an important perspective. One player took a video of the event. He thought it was amazing what they were able to do and did not want to imagine what would have happened if they had not been there to help.

Next, a dozen players lifted the car, and Alan's wife was rescued. Neither of them appeared to have severe injuries. A Deputy Sheriff was unable to arrive until about an hour after the accident. Alan Hardeman expressed his appreciation. He saw no hesitation to help from the team and did not know what they would have done without them!

A few days later, the team visited the home of the Hardeman's daughter where the couple was recovering. They came with flowers, cookies, and cards and presented them with a signed jersey and football. One player couldn't rescue them, but twelve could. Strength came with numbers along with the attitude to help! These players were practicing God's wisdom in helping the needy. *"Blessed is the one who is kind to the needy"* (Proverbs 14:21). The whole team was focused and ready to help. If we will walk with others, share information, and support them in the challenges they face, we too will be a helping team. *"Two are better than one, because they have a good return for their labor: If either of them falls down, one can help the other up. But pity anyone who falls and has no one to help them up"* (Ecclesiastes 4:9-10).

Watch: "Youth football team saves couple in overturned car" at **https://www.youtube.com/watch?v=AmNbPKlACSU**

40,000

What would you do with a ring you find while using a metal detector on a beach? A man found a ring on a beach near St. Augustine, Florida, south of Jacksonville. Next, his integrity or honesty is activated. *"The integrity of the upright guides them, but the unfaithful are destroyed by their duplicity"* (Proverbs 11:3). This man explains integrity with his actions! After he found the ring, he thought it might be worth two thousand dollars. Once he took it to a jeweler for evaluation, he was shocked that its estimated value is 40,000 dollars! "I couldn't believe it," he said.

"That ring has been sitting in my scooter for almost a week."

Then what did he do? Instead of taking it to a resale store, he tried to find the owner by calling forty jewelry stores up and down the coast! Even though that did not seem to work, he still kept the ring. After two weeks, he received a call from an unidentified number. They tried calling him several times, but he wouldn't answer. Finally, he decided to answer as he thought this could be the ring's owner, and it was.

Back to the word *"integrity"*, that means *"being complete"* or *"finished."* The author of 1 Kings used the term to describe the temple. *"And he overlaid the whole house with gold, until all the house was **finished**. Also the whole altar that belonged to the inner sanctuary he overlaid with gold"* (1 Kings 6:22). Being *"finished"* meant the temple was complete.

Integrity also describes moral and ethical completeness or soundness. *"Keep your servant also from willful sins; may they not rule over me. Then I will be **blameless**, innocent of great transgression"* (Psalm 19:13). This was the soundness of Joseph Cook when he found the ring. He was blameless; he was a man of integrity. When a newsperson asked whether he thought about keeping it or selling it, he answered he never thought about selling it or saving it even for a minute. That action was never on his mind. Instead, he intended to return it to the owners, and that is what he did. He is a man of integrity and completeness. "They were pretty happy," he said. "The wife was on a FaceTime call, and she just said, I can't believe it, and then she just started crying." Not only did Joseph contribute to her happiness, but his own as well. *"A generous person will prosper; whoever refreshes others will be refreshed"* (Proverbs 11:25). He said, "It felt really good, I've returned sixty-thousand dollars of stuff this year, but nothing even close to this before." He refreshed the owner and himself by being generous. Let Joseph be our model.

The Story of Firefighters Saving a Man Who Becomes a Firefighter

Remember a time when you felt grateful for something that someone did for you! That "something" is usually meaningful and significant. When one person shared the details of what others did for him, he described them as life-changing for his life was literally saved. "That's not all they saved," he said. "They saved my family the pain of losing me. They saved my little sister's big brother. They saved me the time with my family that I would've never gotten." Does that sound significant? Does that sound meaningful? How was he saved?

Firefighters saved him. He was on the second floor of an apartment complex that was ablaze like a bonfire. This fire was huge! After climbing the ladder and going through the window a firefighter had found him unconscious. He awoke three days later in ICU at the hospital. Nurses told him what happened. He spent the next week in the hospital recovering. His story and the remembrance of what they had done for him motivated him.

Four years later a stranger arrived at the fire station for a "ride-along" (a program designed for observation of a day in the life of a firefighter). At first, no one recognized him until fifteen minutes later he told the major who he was—the person they carried out of an apartment fire four-years before and saved his life! They had given him a great desire! He desired to save others' lives! He had decided to earn his firefighter's degree.[136]

The Story of Zacchaeus

Two thousand years ago another man's life was saved. No one would have anything to do with him. He was an outcast because he was a hated tax collector. No one would expect the rabbi, the teacher, to go to his home and eat with him. His name was Zacchaeus and since he was so short, he climbed a sycamore-fig tree to see Jesus among the crowd. *"When Jesus reached the spot, he looked up and said to him, 'Zacchaeus, come down immediately. I must stay at your house today' So, he came down at once and welcomed him gladly."* Then we find him saying something very interesting. His life was being changed by Jesus. Jesus coming to his home was already motivating kindness in him. He said, *"Look, Lord! Here and now I give half of my possessions to the poor, and if I have cheated anybody out of anything, I will pay back four times the amount"* (Luke 19:5-6, 8). Zacchaeus was showing he was a changed man, a man of compassion. Jesus had saved this outcast's life. Would this be the "something" Zacchaeus could remember with gratitude? When we think back on events that others have done for us, it brings out the best in us. It happened to the man saved by firefighters and it happened to Zacchaeus. *"For the Son of Man came to seek and to save the lost"* (Luke 19:10).

Jesus had a reputation for being compassionate and kind toward people. He cared about people. When he looked at people, he pictured them as being harassed and helpless like sheep without a shepherd. He saw hurting people! *"He said to his disciples, 'The harvest is plentiful but the workers are few. Ask the Lord of the harvest, therefore, to send out workers into his harvest field'"* (Matthew 9:37-38.) He saw the need for more kind, compassionate workers!

The Story of the Apostle Paul

One man remembered a man who saved his life two thousand years ago, rescuing him from a destructive lifestyle. If this man could change from a vicious lifestyle to a lifestyle of gratitude, service, and love, so can anyone. He described himself as a persecutor, a violent man, and the worst of sinners. Why did he describe himself as a violent man? Hunting for people who were disciples of Jesus, forcing them to deny Jesus or face imprisonment or execution, is why he considered himself violent. He separated families with imprisonment or death when they refused to deny Jesus. He says, *"Many a time I went from one synagogue to another to have them punished, and I tried to force them to blaspheme. In my obsession against them, I even went to foreign cities to persecute them"* (Acts 26:11). Who or what could change such a vicious man?

The kindness and love he saw in a man who cared about people motivated him to live a life of love. He describes his new way of life with these words he wrote to a young man named Timothy. *"You, however, know all about my teaching, my way of life, my purpose, faith, patience, love, endurance, persecutions, sufferings"* (2 Timothy 3:10-11). His new life caused him to face persecution rather than be the perpetrator. Kindness has a strange response at times, like ugly violence, but usually appreciation. His lifestyle, in his words, *"In everything I did, I showed you that by this kind of hard work we must help the weak, remembering the words the Lord Jesus himself said: 'It is more blessed to give than to receive'"* (Acts 20:35).

The kindness and love of Jesus changed Paul's life! Paul writes, *"Christ Jesus came into the world to save sinners—of whom*

I am the worst" (1 Timothy 1:15). He describes patience and kindness as attributes of love, which is what Jesus had for him (1 Corinthians 13:4). Jesus' love for him, his mercy, and compassion changed his life from violence to kindness (read Titus 3:4-5). Treating people as Jesus did was his desire. He wrote, *"Be imitators of me as I am of Christ"* (1 Corinthians 11:1). Paul describes Jesus' disciples as *"God's handiwork, created in Christ Jesus to do good works"* (Ephesians 2:10). Saved, or delivered from his life of violence and sin meant he writes being *"devoted to doing what is good"* (Titus 3:8). Grasping the depth of Jesus' love for him compelled him to live, not for himself, but for Jesus—to live a life of love (2 Corinthians 5:14, Ephesians 5:2).

Struck blind while hunting down disciples of Jesus to force them to deny their loyalty to Jesus or be imprisoned or even put to death gave him, in a sense, new life (Acts 26:11). He was on the road to Damascus when a bright light from heaven blinded him. Jesus spoke to him, saying, *"Saul, Saul, why do you persecute me?" "Who are you, Lord?" Saul asked. "I am Jesus, whom you are persecuting,"* he replied. *"Now get up and go into the city, and you will be told what you must do"* (Acts 9:4-6). So, he went to Damascus. Blind, praying and fasting for three days, Ananias, a disciple of Jesus, came to him and said, *"And now what are you waiting for? Get up, be baptized and wash your sins away, calling on his name"* (Acts 22:16). At that moment, he was saved, becoming a disciple of Jesus.

He could see again, but he saw life differently. He now had a new life. He was a new creation. *"If anyone is in Christ, the new creation has come: The old has gone, the new is here"* (2 Corinthians 5:17). All the havoc and harm he brought to people is now forgiven, washed away! He was a changed man. Instead of persecuting people, he began telling people how much Jesus loved them as he lived a life of love himself.

When he told people how to become compassionate, kind disciples of Jesus, he tied it directly to what Jesus had done for them. *"Or don't you know that all of us who were baptized into Christ Jesus were baptized into his death? We were therefore buried with him through baptism into death in order that, just as Christ was raised from the dead through the glory of the Father, we too may live a new life"* (Romans 6:3-4). And just how much does he say Jesus loves us? *"You see, at just the right time, when we were still powerless, Christ died for the ungodly. Very rarely will anyone die for a righteous person, though for a good person someone might possibly dare to die. But God demonstrates his own love for us in this: While we were still sinners, Christ died for us"* (Romans 5:6-8). A righteous person is just and fair, whereas a good person is just, fair, and generous. But Jesus died, demonstrating his love for the ungodly.

We are all in the ungodly category, yet Jesus was still willing to die for us. That makes us, in Jesus' view most valuable people! So, the apostle John writes, *"This is how we know what love is: Jesus Christ laid down his life for us"* (1 John 3:16). In summarizing Jesus' life, Peter said, *"he went around doing good"* (Acts 10:38). Paul was changed to do good, and let's do the same! Let's help people win a victory over diabetes!

About the Authors

KEN ELLIS has successfully lived with Type 1 Diabetes for sixty-four+ years. He was diagnosed with Type 1 Diabetes during the fall of his first-grade year. For more than thirty years, he has facilitated community Diabetes support groups, presented monthly Diabetes seminars, and helped hundreds of people manage their diabetes in several states. He is now a retired minister after serving for forty-two years.

Ken is a participant in the 50-year medalist research study and has been awarded the 50-year medal from the world-renowned Joslin Diabetes Center, which is affiliated with Harvard Medical School in Boston. This award represents his accomplishment in Diabetes management for fifty years.

DEB ELLIS is an administrative assistant. She is experienced in corporate, government, and school responsibilities. More importantly, she is Ken's wife of almost fifty years, helping him with diabetes educational seminars, meal planning, and giving positive support for his diabetes management!

Contact: www.wisdomfordiabetes.org
Email: ken@wisdomfordiabetes.org

Bible Versions

All Scripture quotations, unless otherwise indicated, are taken from the Holy Bible, New International Version®, NIV®. Copyright ©1973, 1978, 1984, 2011 by Biblica, Inc.™ Used by permission of Zondervan. All rights reserved worldwide. www.zondervan.com The "NIV" and "New International Version" are trademarks registered in the United States Patent and Trademark Office by Biblica, Inc.™

Scriptures taken from the Holy Bible, New International Reader's Version®, NIrV® Copyright © 1995, 1996, 1998 by Biblica, Inc.™ Used by permission of Zondervan. www.zondervan.com The "NIrV" and "New International Reader's Version" are trademarks registered in the United States Patent and Trademark Office by Biblica, Inc.™

Scripture taken from the New Century Version®. Copyright © 2005 by Thomas Nelson. Used by permission. All rights reserved.

"New Revised Standard Version Bible: Anglicized Edition, copyright 1989, 1995, Division of Christian Education of the National Council of the Churches of Christ in the United States of America. Used by permission. All rights re-served."

Scripture taken from the New King James Version®. Copyright © 1982 by Thomas Nelson. Used by permission. All rights reserved.

"Scripture quotations taken from the New American Standard Bible®, Copyright © 1960, 1962, 1963, 1968, 1971, 1972, 1973, 1975, 1977, 1995 by The Lockman Foundation

Used by permission." (**www.Lockman.org**)

Bibliography

Michael Bliss, **The Discovery of Insulin** (The University of Chicago Press, Chicago, 1982).

Michael Breus, Ph.D. and Debra Fulgham Bruce Ph.D., **The Sleep Doctor's Diet Plan: Simple Rules for Losing Weight While You Sleep** (Rodale Books, 2012).

Dr. Will Bulsiewicz **Fiber Fueled: The Plant-Based Gut Health Program for Losing Weight, Restoring Your Health, and Optimizing Your Microbiome** (Avery 2020).

Dr. Sheri R. Colberg, **Diabetes and Keeping Fit** (by John Wiley & Sons, Inc., Hoboken, New Jersey, 2018).

Ken Ellis, **7 Biblical Ways for Healthy Living, 2020.**

Ken Ellis, **The Way of Wisdom for Diabetes, 2016.**

Mark Ehrman and Sara Mednick, **Take a Nap! Change Your Life.** (Workman Publishing Company May 2018).

Robert A. Emmons, Ph.D., **Thanks! How Practicing Gratitude Can Make You Happier** (Houghton Mifflin Company, New York, 2007).

Nichole Dandrea-Russert RDN **The Fiber Effect: Stop Counting Calories and Start Counting Fiber for Better Health** (Hatherleigh Press; 1st edition 2021).

Dr. Jason Fung, **The Diabetes Code: Prevent and Reverse Type 2 Diabetes Naturally** (Greystone Books Ltd., 2018).

Johann Hari. **Magic Pill: The Extraordinary Benefits and Disturbing Risks of the New Weight-Loss Drugs** (Crown, 2024).

Jessie Inchauspe, **Glucose Revolution: The Life-Changing Power of Balancing Your Blood Sugar** (Simon Element, New York, 2022).

Dr. James Levine, **Move a Little, Lose a Lot: Use N.E.A.T.* Science to: Burn 2,100 Calories a Week at the Office, Be Smarter in as Little as 3 Hours, Reduce Fatigue by 65%, Extend Your Lifespan by 4 Years** (Harmony; 1st edition 2009).

Dr. James Levine, **Get Up!: Why Your Chair is Killing You and What You Can Do About It** (Griffin 2014).

Dr. Marty Makary. **Blind Spots: When Medicine Gets It Wrong, and What It Means for Our Health** (Bloomsbury Publishing, 2024).

Dr. Casey Means and Calley Means, **Good Energy: The Surprising Connection Between Metabolism and Limitless Health** (Penguin Publishing Group, 2023).

Jordin Ruben and Dr. Josh Axe, **Essential Fasting: 12 Benefits of Intermittent Fasting** (DESTINY IMAGE® PUBLISHERS, INC., 2020).

Dr. Rob Thompson, Dana Carpender, **The Insulin Resistance Solution: Reverse Pre-Diabetes, Repair Your Metabolism, Shed Belly Fat, Prevent Diabetes** (2023).

Joan Vernikos, Ph.D, **Sitting Kills, Moving Heals: How Everyday Movement Will Prevent Pain, Illness, and Early Death—and Exercise Alone Won't"** (Quill Driver Books; 1st edition 2011).

Brian Wansink, Ph.D., **Mindless Eating: Why We Eat More Than We Think** (New York: Bantam Dell, 2006).

Endnotes

1   Texas Police Make Odd Withdrawal from ATM: A Man Who Was Trapped Inside, Colin Dwyer, **https://www.npr.org/sections/thetwo-way/2017/07/13/537043822/texas-police-make-odd-withdrawal-from-atm-a-man-who-was-trapped-inside** (Accessed August 2023)

2   Richard Beaser, MD, ed., Joslin Diabetes Deskbook: A Guide for Primary Care Providers (Boston: Joslin Diabetes Center, 2014), 4, 5.

3   Michael Bliss, The Discovery of Insulin (Chicago: The University of Chicago Press, 1982), 161, 164.

4   Forester McClatchey Banting—The Man, the Myth, the Legend **https://beyondtype1.org/banting-the-man-the-myth-the-legend/** (Accessed August 2024).

5   Michael Bliss, The Discovery of Insulin (Chicago: The University of Chicago Press, 1982), 112, 243.

6   Dan J. Weinert, Nutrition and muscle protein synthesis: a descriptive review (August 2009) **https://www.ncbi.nlm.nih.gov/pmc/articles/PMC2732256/** (Accessed August 2023).

7   Jason Fung, MD, The Diabetes Code: Prevent and Reverse Type 2 Diabetes Naturally (Greystone Books Ltd., 2018), 80.

8   Matthew T. Draelos, MD, Health Tips **https://www.draelosmetabolic.com/dr-draelos-health-tips** (Accessed March 2019).

9   Incretin Hormone, Diabetes Self-management, (March 13, 2009) **https://www.diabetesselfmanagement.com/diabetes-resources/definitions/incretin-hormone/** (Accessed March 2019).

10   Jennie Brand-Miller, PhD, Kaye Foster-Powell, and Rick Mendosa, What Makes My Blood Glucose Go Up . . . and Down?: And 101 Other Frequently Asked Questions About Your Blood Glucose Levels (New York: Marlowe & Company, 2003), 173-182.

11   Barbara Rolls, PhD, Salad and Satiety: Energy Density and Portion Size of a First-Course Salad Affect Energy Intake at Lunch, Department of Nutritional Sciences, The Pennsylvania State University, **http://www.ncbi.nlm.nih.gov/pubmed/15389416** - October, 2004 (Accessed September 2024)

12   Richard Beaser, MD, ed., Joslin Diabetes Deskbook: A Guide for Primary Care Providers (Boston: Joslin Diabetes Center, 2014), 112.

13   Robert A. Emmons, Thanks: How Practicing Gratitude Can Make You Happier (New York: Houghton Mifflin Company, 2007), 27, 32–33.

14   Rob Thompson M.D. and Dana Carpender, The Insulin Resistance Solution: Reverse Pre-Diabetes, Repair Your Metabolism, Shed Belly Fat, Prevent Diabetes

15   Sheri R. Colberg, Diabetes and Keeping Fit For Dummies (pp. 189-190). Wiley. Kindle Edition.

16   Exercise intensity: How to measure it, https://www.mayoclinic.org/healthy-lifestyle/fitness/in-depth/exercise-intensity/art-20046887 (Accessed July 2019).

17   Standing for healthier lives—literally, Francisco Lopez-Jimenez, MD, Mayo Clinic. **https://academic.oup.com/eurheartj/article/36/39/2650/2398350** (Accessed May 2018).

18   Researchers say to stand up, sit less and move more. Carolina Storrs, CNN August 6, 2015, **http://www.cnn.com/2015/08/06/health/how-to-move-more/index.html** (Accessed May 2018).

19   Sheri R. Colberg, Diabetes and Keeping Fit For Dummies (pp. 189-190). Wiley. Kindle Edition.

20   'I Have Terminal Brain Cancer. I Just Did An Ironman To Inspire My 5-Year-Old,' Jenny Haward, **https://www.newsweek.com/i-have-terminal-brain-cancer-i-just-did-ironman-inspire-daughter-1538800** (Accessed August, 2023).

21   Walter Willett, MD, Eat, Drink, and Weigh Less: A Flexible and Delicious Way to Shrink your Waist Without Going Hungry (New York: Tante Malka, Inc., 2006), 67.

22   Drinking Water May Cut Risk of High Blood Sugar, Charlene Laino, **http://diabetes.webmd.com/news/20110630/drinking-water-may-cut-risk-of-high-blood-sugar** (Accessed March 12, 2018).

23   Barbara Rolls, Ph.D., The Volumetrics Eating Plan: Techniques and Recipes for Feeling Full on Fewer Calories (New York: HarperCollins Publishers, 2005), 10.

24   Artificial sweeteners: sugar-free, but at what cost? Holly Strawbridge **https://www.health.harvard.edu/blog/artificial-sweeteners-sugar-free-but-at-what-cost-2017165030** (Accessed March 16, 2018).

25   Urine Color, Mayo Clinic Staff, **https://www.mayoclinic.org/
      diseases-conditions/urine-color/symptoms-causes/syc-
      20367333** (Accessed March 12, 2018)

26   Water and Stress Reduction: Sipping Stress Away, Gina
      Shaw, **http://www.webmd.com/diet/features/water-stress-
      reduction** (Accessed March 12, 2018).

27   Robert K. Cooper, Ph.D., Flip the Switch Lose the Weight:
      Proven Strategies to Fuel Your Metabolism & Burn Fat 24 Hours
      a Day (New York: Rodale Inc., 2005), 78-79.

28   Brian Wansink, Ph.D., Mindless Eating: Why We Eat More Than
      We Think (New York: Bantam Dell, 2006), 189.

29   Dr. Marty Makary. Blind Spots: When Medicine Gets It Wrong,
      and What It Means for Our Health (p. 63). Bloomsbury
      Publishing. Kindle Edition.

30   G. A. Soliman, "Dietary Cholesterol and the Lack of Evidence in
      Cardiovascular Disease," Nutrients 10, no. 6 (June 2018): 780.

31   Dr. Jason Fung. The Diabetes Code: 2 (The Code Series) (p.
      219). Greystone Books. Kindle Edition.

32   Mark Ehrman and Sara Mednick, Take a Nap! Change Your Life.
      (pp. 23-28). Workman Publishing Company May 2018. Kindle
      Edition.

33   The Health Benefits of Napping: Resting Can Help Reduce
      Stress and Protect Immune System, Lecia Bushak, Medical
      Daily, February 10, 2015, **http://www.medicaldaily.com/
      health-benefits-napping-resting-can-help-reduce-stress-
      and-protect-immune-system-321580** (Accessed August
      2019).

34   How to get the most out of napping, Micah Dorfner, **https://newsnetwork.mayoclinic.org/discussion/how-to-get-the-most-out-of-napping/** March 28, 2018 (Accessed August 2019).

35   Jessie Inchauspe, Glucose Revolution: The Life-Changing Power of Balancing Your Blood Sugar (p. 92). S&S/Simon Element. Kindle Edition.

36   Broccoli Nutrition Helps Battle Cancer, Osteoporosis & Weight Gain, Jillian Levy, CHHC October 3, 2022, https://draxe.com/nutrition/broccoli-nutrition/

37   Omega-3 Fatty Acids: Benefits for the Heart, Brain, Joints & More, Dr. Josh Axe May 2, 2024, **https://draxe.com/nutrition/omega-3-fatty-acids/**

38   Top Foods High in Omega-3s, Medically Reviewed by Jabeen Begum, MD. **https://www.webmd.com/diet/foods-high-in-omega-3**

39   Break the Cycle of Yo-Yo Dieting, Jennifer Hubert, DO January 9, 2018 https://blog.providence.org/healthcalling/break-the-cycle-of-yo-yo-dieting

40   Rob Thompson, M.D., and Dana Carpender. The Insulin Resistance Solution: Reverse Pre-Diabetes, Repair Your Metabolism, Shed Belly Fat, Prevent Diabetes (p. 62). Quarto Publishing Group USA. Kindle Edition.

41   Ibid (p. 62).

42   Remembering Ida Keeling, Who Set Track Records into Her 100s, Nadia Neophytou Sept 15, 2021 (Accessed August 2023).

43   Osama Hamdy and Sheri R. Colberg, Sheri R, The Diabetes Breakthrough: Based on a Scientifically Proven Plan to Lose Weight and Cut Medications (Kindle Location 2950). Harlequin. Kindle Edition.

44   Ozempic for Weight Loss: How Does It Work and Who Can Use It?, Alyssa Billingsley, PharmD and Christina Aungst, PharmD, Updated on April 26, 2023

45   Mounjaro More Effective Than Ozempic for Weight Loss, New Research Shows, Victoria Stokes, August 2, 2023

46   'Ozempic Face': What It Is And How To Treat It, Amy Mackelden. **https://www.forbes.com/health/weight-loss/ozempic-face/**

47   **https://revitalizeweightloss.com/blog/semaglutide-vs-intermittent-fasting/**

48   Does Ozempic Make You Lose More Muscle? June 20, 2024. **https://www.brgeneral.org/news-blog/2024/june/does-ozempic-make-you-lose-more-muscle-/** (Accessed September 9 2024).

49   Preserve your muscle mass, Harvard Health Publishing – Harvard Medical School, February, 2016, **https://www.health.harvard.edu/staying-healthy/preserve-your-muscle-mass#:~:text=Most%20men%20will%20lose%20about,risk%20of%20falls%20and%20fractures** (Accessed August 18 2020).

50   Age-related changes in gait, balance, and strength parameters: A cross-sectional study **https://journals.plos.org/plosone/article?id=10.1371/journal.pone.0310764**

51   Mayo Clinic study: What standing on one leg can tell you, Rhoda Madson, October 23, 2024 **https://newsnetwork.mayoclinic.org/discussion/mayo-clinic-study-what-standing-on-one-leg-can-tell-you/**

52   How long can you stand on one leg? What it says about your health. Laura Baisas, October 24, 2024, **https://www.popsci.com/health/standing-on-one-leg-aging/**

53   Ibid. (Accessed November 7 2024).

54   Johann Hari. Magic Pill: The Extraordinary Benefits and Disturbing Risks of the New Weight-Loss Drugs (p. 84). Crown. Kindle Edition.

55   Ozempic and Muscle Loss: Preserving Muscle Mass on GLP-1Medications. **https://www.hingehealth.com/resources/articles/ozempic-muscle-loss/** (Accessed September 9 2024)

56   Could the Timing of When You Eat, Be Just as Important as What You Eat? Science Daily, January 29, 2013, Source: Brigham and Women's Hospital. **http://www.sciencedaily.com/releases/2013/01/130129080620.htm**   (Accessed August 2019)

57   Dietary Fat Acutely Increases Glucose Concentrations and Insulin Requirements in Patients With Type 1 Diabetes, **https://www.ncbi.nlm.nih.gov/pmc/articles/PMC3609492/** (Accessed September 2024).

58   Ibid.

59   Time-restricted feeding study shows promise in helping people shed body fat, Adam Pope, January 09, 2017, **https://www.uab.edu/news/health/item/7869-time-restricted-feeding-study-shows-promise-in-helping-people-shed-body-fat** (Accessed August 2019).

60   Stages of Fasting by Hour and Fat Burning Stage Fasting, June 5, 2022, https://kompanionapp.com/en/fasting-fat-burning-stage/

61   Adiponectin – Secret Weight Loss Weapon, Dr. Aarthi Maria, 10 Oct 2019, **https://www.baymedicalaesthetics.com.au/adiponectin-secret-weight-loss-weapon**

62   How to Increase Adinopectin Naturally, **https://fivejourneys.com/how-to-increase-adiponectin-the-fat-burning-hormone**

63   How Much Sleep Do I Need?, **https://www.cdc.gov/sleep/about_sleep/how_much_sleep.html** (Accessed August 2019).

64   How Much Sleep Do Fitbit Users Really Get? A New Study Finds Out, Danielle Kosecki, June 29, 2017, **https://blog.fitbit.com/sleep-study/** (Accessed August 2019).

65   Drowsy Driving: Asleep at the Wheel, **https://www.cdc.gov/features/dsdrowsydriving/index.html** (Accessed August 2019).

66   Michael Breus. The Sleep Doctor's Diet Plan: Simple Rules for Losing Weight While You Sleep (p. 8). Potter/Ten Speed/Harmony/Rodale. Kindle Edition.

67   Sleep and Metabolism: An Overview, 2010, **https://www.ncbi.nlm.nih.gov/pmc/articles/PMC2929498/** (Accessed August 2019)

68   Breus, 9-10.

69   Breus, 44.

70   Sleep and Metabolism: An Overview, Int J Endocrinol. 2010. **https://www.ncbi.nlm.nih.gov/pmc/articles/PMC2929498/** (Accessed August 2019).

71   Breus, 28-29.

72   Maximising Your Melatonin, **https://instituteofhealthsciences.com/maximising-your-melatonin/** (Accessed August 2019).

73   Melatonin, **https://www.webmd.com/vitamins/ai/ingredientmono-940/melatonin** (Accessed August 2019).

[74] Top 20 Ways to Fall Asleep Fast! Dr. Josh Axe, **https://draxe.com/cant-sleep/** (Accessed August 2019).

[75] Robert A. Emmons, Thanks: How Practicing Gratitude Can Make You Happier (New York: Houghton Mifflin Company, 2007), 27. Emmons, 32–33.

[76] Stephen Post, Why Good Things Happen to Good People: The Exciting New Research That Proves the Link Between Doing Good and Living a Longer, Healthier, Happier Life (New York: Broadway Books, 2007), 28, 30.

[77] Personal Accounts of the Negative and Adaptive Psychosocial Experiences of People With Diabetes in the Second Diabetes Attitudes, Wishes and Needs (DAWN2) Study, Heather L. Stuckey, Diabetes Care September, 2014 **http://care.diabetesjournals.org/content/37/9/2466** (Accessed August 2019).

[78] Richard Beaser, MD, ed., Joslin Diabetes Deskbook: A Guide for Primary Care Providers (Boston: Joslin Diabetes Center, 2014), 437-440.

[79] John Walsh, PA, CDE, Using Insulin: Everything You Need for Success with Insulin (San Diego: Torrey Pines Press, 2003), 220.

[80] Loneliness is universal: Boca students' message that nobody should eat alone is heard worldwide, **https://www.sun-sentinel.com/local/broward/fl-boca-raton-we-dine-together-goes-viral-20170417-story.html** (Accessed August 2019).

81   A Bike Accident Left This ER Doctor Paralyzed. Now He's Back
      At Work, Chris Bentley, and Jeremy Hobson, (June 06, 2018),
      **https://www.wbur.org/hereandnow/2018/06/06/doctor-
      paralyzed-mayo-clinic** (Accessed March 2019).

82   George G. Ritchie, and Elizabeth Sherrill, Return from
      Tomorrow (Grand Rapids, MI: Baker Publishing Group, 1978,
      2007), 131..

83   US man clings to glider after taking off unsecured to craft,
      Bryce Luff, PerthNow, (November 27, 2018) **https://www.
      perthnow.com.au/news/europe/us-man-clings-to-glider-
      after-taking-off-unsecured-to-craft-ng-b881033549z**
      (Accessed March 2019).

84   Gary Arsham, MD, and Ernest Lowe, Diabetes: A Guide
      to Living Well (Alexandria, Virginia: American Diabetes
      Association, 2004), 183-184.

85   Joseph P. Napora, PhD, Stress-Free Diabetes: Your Guide
      to Health and Happiness (Alexandria, Virginia: American
      Diabetes Association, 2010), 1–2.

86   Police officer stuck behind a tortoise posts video
      of his encounter **https://www.youtube.com/
      watch?v=dUEz6AmUPPQ**

87   Minnesota man rescued after 4 days trapped under fallen
      tree, The Associated Press, **https://abcnews.go.com/US/
      wireStory/minnesota-man-rescued-days-trapped-fallen-
      tree-72815611** (Accessed October 14, 2020).

88   Minnesota man trapped underneath a fallen tree for 4 days
      is rescued, Minyvonne Burke, Sept. 5, 2020, **https://www.
      nbcnews.com/news/us-news/minnesota-man-trapped-
      underneath-fallen-tree-4-days-rescued-n1239412**

89   Chris Feudtner, M.D., Bittersweet: Diabetes, Insulin, and the Transformation of Illness (Chapel Hill: The University of North Carolina Press, 2003), 52.

90   Michael Bliss, The Making of Modern Medicine: Turning Points in the Treatment of Disease (Chicago: The University of Chicago Press, 2011), 76.

91   David O. Woodbury, "Please Save My Son" Reader's Digest, (volume 82, number 490, February, 1963), 157-162.

92   "Miracle Boy" Wakes From Coma Day Before Parents Pull The Plug On Life Support, May 7, 2018, **https://alt1037dfw.radio.com/blogs/miracle-boy-wakes-coma-day-parents-pull-plug-life-support** (Accessed August 2019).

93   Teen heart transplant patient finds miracle wrapped in delay, August 29, 2014, **https://www.khou.com/article/news/health/teen-heart-transplant-patient-finds-miracle-wrapped-in-delay/259142526** (Accessed August 2019).

94   Henry Dolger, M.D. and Bernard Seeman, How to Live with Diabetes (New York: Pyramid Books, 1958), 103.

95   Dolger, 84.

96   Woman Is Brought To Tears By Thank You Note After Act Of Kindness In Grocery Store, January 11, 2019, **https://www.sunnyskyz.com/good-news/3170/Woman-Is-Brought-To-Tears-By-Thank-You-Note-After-Act-Of-Kindness-In-Grocery-Store** (Accessed August 2019).

97   Personal Accounts of the Negative and Adaptive Psychosocial
      Experiences of People With Diabetes in the Second Diabetes
      Attitudes, Wishes and Needs (DAWN2) Study, Heather
      L. Stuckey, Diabetes Care September 2014 **http://care.
      diabetesjournals.org/content/37/9/2466** (Accessed May
      2018).

98   Second Diabetes Attitudes, Wishes and Needs (DAWN2) Study,
      Heather L. Stuckey.

99   Gary Arsham, MD, and Ernest Lowe, Diabetes: A Guide
      to Living Well (Alexandria, Virginia: American Diabetes
      Association, 2004), 15.

100   Catherine Cox, The Fight to Survive (New York: Kaplan
      Publishing, 2009), 113–14.

101   Michael Bliss, The Discovery of Insulin (Chicago: The
      University of Chicago Press, 1982), 152.

102   A soldier says a stranger's Christmas card got him through
      Vietnam. He just met the sender, November 17, 2018, **https://
      www.wivb.com/news/national/a-soldier-says-a-strangers-
      christmas-card-got-him-through-vietnam-he-just-met-the-
      sender/** (Accessed August 2019).

103   Richard Jackson, MD, and Amy Tenderich, Know Your
      Numbers, Outlive Your Diabetes: Five Essential Health Factors
      You Can Master to Enjoy a Long and Healthy Life (New York:
      Marlowe & Company, 2007), 104, 107.

104   **https://diabetes.org/about-diabetes/statistics/about-
      diabetes** August, 2024 (Accessed August 2024).

105   The Origin of the 10,000-Steps-Per-Day Goal, Natalie
      Shoemaker, **http://bigthink.com/ideafeed/the-origin-of-the-
      10000-steps-per-day-goal** (Accessed May, 2018).

106   The Surprising Number of Steps Americans Really Take Each Day, Sarah Klein, Health, July 13, 2017, **http://www.health.com/fitness/number-of-steps-americans-take-daily** (Accessed May, 2018).

107   Adult Obesity Facts, **https://www.cdc.gov/obesity/data/adult.html** (Accessed May 2018).

108   Walking, **https://www.cdc.gov/physicalactivity/walking/index.htm** (Accessed May 2018).

109   How Many Steps/Day Are Enough? Preliminary Pedometer Indices for Public Health, Catrine Tudor-Locke, Ph.D., and David R. Bassett, Jr., Ph.D., **https://www.renevanmaarsseveen.nl/wp-content/uploads/overig6/how%20many%20steps%20are%20enough%20-%20catrine%20tudor%20locke.pdf** (Accessed August 19, 2020).

110   Walking 10,000 steps/day or more reduces blood pressure and sympathetic nerve activity in mild essential hypertension. **https://www.ncbi.nlm.nih.gov/pubmed/11131268** (Accessed May 2018).

111   Increasing daily walking improves glucose tolerance in overweight women. **https://www.ncbi.nlm.nih.gov/pubmed/14507493** (Accessed May, 2018).

112   Means, Casey; Means, Calley. Good Energy: The Surprising Connection Between Metabolism and Limitless Health (p. 219). Penguin Publishing Group. Kindle Edition.

113   https://drhyman.com/blogs/content/what-the-heck-are-mitochondria#:~:text=Mitochondria%20are%20where%20metabolism%20happens,VERY%20sensitive%20and%20easily%20damaged.

114   Metabolic Flexibility and Its Impact on Health Outcomes. https://www.mayoclinicproceedings.org/article/S0025-6196(22)00042-8/fulltext

115   Rob Thompson M.D. and Dana Carpender, The Insulin Resistance Solution: Reverse Pre-Diabetes, Repair Your Metabolism, Shed Belly Fat, Prevent Diabetes

116   Sheri R. Colberg, Diabetes and Keeping Fit for Dummies (pp. 189-190). Wiley. Kindle Edition.

117   "How exercise -- interval training in particular -- helps your mitochondria stave off old age." ScienceDaily. ScienceDaily, 7 March 2017.

118   Mayo Clinic: Mitochondrial Health – Keeping Your Tiny Powerhouses in Tip-Top Shape. https://www.thorne.com/take-5-daily/article/mayo-clinic-mitochondrial-health-keeping-your-tiny-powerhouses-in-tip-top-shape#:~:text=Although%20more%20

119   Effects of Physical Activity and Weight Loss on Skeletal Muscle Mitochondria and Relationship With Glucose Control in Type 2 Diabetes. https://diabetesjournals.org/diabetes/article/56/8/2142/14426/Effects-of-Physical-Activity-and-Weight-Loss-on

120   Mayo Clinic: Mitochondrial Health – Keeping Your Tiny Powerhouses in Tip-Top Shape. https://www.thorne.com/take-5-daily/article/mayo-clinic-mitochondrial-health-keeping-your-tiny-powerhouses-in-tip-top-shape

121   Metabolic Flexibility and Its Impact on Health Outcomes. https://www.mayoclinicproceedings.org/article/S0025-6196(22)00042-8/fulltext

122   Stages of Fasting by Hour and Fat Burning Stage Fasting, June 5, 2022, https:// kompanionapp.com/en/fasting-fat-burning-stage/

123   https://www.timeline.com/blog/the-importance-of-mitochondrial-health-a-user-guide? by Jen Scheinman, MS, RDN, CDN

124   Michael Breus. The Sleep Doctor's Diet Plan: Simple Rules for Losing Weight While You Sleep (p. 8). Potter/ Ten Speed/ Harmony/ Rodale. Kindle Edition.

125   Sleep and Metabolism: An Overview, 2010, https:// www.ncbi.nlm.nih.gov/pmc/articles/PMC2929498/ (Accessed August 2019) (Accessed August 2019)

126   Breus, 9-10.

127   https://www.mitoq.com/journal/how-does-sleep-affect-mitochondria

128   Mitochondria (Part 6): Change Your Lifestyle, Change Your Mitochondria. Dr. Maya Kuczma. https://integrative.ca/blog/mitochondria-part-6-change-your-lifestyle-change-your-mitochondria

129   A father and his sons cut wood to fill 80 trucks. Then they brought it to homes that needed heat, Caitlin Huson, December 21, 2018, https://www.washingtonpost.com/lifestyle/2018/12/21/father-his-sons-cut-wood-fill-trucks-then-they-brought-it-homes-that-needed-heat/?noredirect=on (Accessed August 2019).

130 107-Year-Old Is The World's Oldest Barber And He's Still Cutting Hair Full Time, October 14, 2018, **https://www.sunnyskyz.com/good-news/3040/107-Year-Old-Is-The-World-039-s-Oldest-Barber-And-He-039-s-Still-Cutting-Hair-Full-Time** (Accessed August 2019).

131 99-year-old man walks 6 miles a day to visit his wife in the hospital, proving true love does exist, August 31, 2018, **https://www.cbsnews.com/news/99-year-old-man-luther-younger-walks-six-miles-a-day-to-visit-his-wife-in-the-hospital-rochester-new-york/** (Accessed August 2019).

132 Albert Lexie, the shoe-shiner who donated $200K to UPMC Children's Hospital, has died, Bob Batz Jr. Pittsburgh Post-Gazette, October 16, 2018, **https://www.post-gazette.com/news/obituaries/2018/10/16/albert-lexie-children-s-hospital-pittsburgh-shoe-shiner-monessen-obituary-foundation/stories/201810160158** (Accessed August 2019).

133 Woman's New Year's Resolution Saves A Stranger's Life, June 14, 2018, **https://www.sunnyskyz.com/good-news/2855/Woman-039-s-New-Year-039-s-Resolution-Saves-A-Stranger-039-s-Life** (Accessed August 2019).

134 Florida woman who survived Holocaust turns 100, throws first pitch at Yankees-Rays game: 'Really wonderfull,' Gretchen Eichenberg Fox News, May 8, 2023, **https://www.foxnews.com/lifestyle/florida-woman-survived-holocaust-turns-100-throws-first-pitch-yankees-rays-game-really-wonderful**

135 Boise youth football team meets with couple they helped rescue from overturned car, Michael Katz, Idaho Statesman, May 30 and June 1, 2018, **https://www.idahostatesman.com/latest-news/article212236279.html** (Accessed August 2019).

[136] Metro Rescue Victim To Become Firefighter, Christy Lewis, Oklahoma City News9, February 23, 2018, **http://www.news9.com/story/37580818/metro-rescue-victim-to-become-firefighter** (Accessed August 2019).